Integrative Endocrinology

T0229681

This book explains the treatment of endocrine disorders using natural therapies. Donald Beans provides the reader with everything there is to know to treat endocrine disorders without hormones. This book outlines the function of the endocrine glands and the testing of their function, including clinical laboratory evaluation and bedside diagnosis. This is the first book to include the entire endocrine system and many natural therapies in one text, thus allowing the practitioner an unprecedented insight into endocrine treatment. *Integrative Endocrinology* discusses, in depth, the fundamental philosophical difference between hormone replacement therapy and integrative endocrinology.

Natural therapies include acupuncture, gland cell therapy, homeopathy, herbal medicine, and a number of other methods. This book is of great value to health professionals, students, and scholars in integrative medicine, alternative medicine, and endocrinology. It is also valuable as a self-help handbook for the motivated non-professional.

Donald R. Beans is a state licensed and nationally certified acupuncturist and certified classical homeopath with a doctorate in iridology and nutrition.

Integrative Endocrinology
The Rhythms of Life

Donald R. Beans

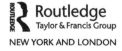
Routledge
Taylor & Francis Group

NEW YORK AND LONDON

First published 2010
by Routledge
711 Third Ave, New York, NY 10017

Simultaneously published in the UK
by Routledge
2 Park Square, Milton Park, Abingdon, Oxon OX14 4RN

Routledge is an imprint of the Taylor & Francis Group, an informa business

© 2010 Donald R. Beans

Typeset in Sabon by
Book Now Ltd, London

All rights reserved. No part of this book may be reprinted or reproduced or utilised in any form or by any electronic, mechanical, or other means, now known or hereafter invented, including photocopying and recording, or in any information storage or retrieval system, without permission in writing from the publishers.

Trademark Notice: Product or corporate names may be trademarks or registered trademarks, and are used only for identification and explanation without intent to infringe.

Disclaimer: Taylor & Francis do not take responsibility for the practices or treatments described in this book.

Library of Congress Cataloging-in-Publication Data
Beans, Donald R.
Integrative endocrinology: the rhythms of life / Donald R. Beans.
       p. cm.
Includes bibliographical references and index.
1. Endocrine glands—Diseases—Alternative treatment. I. Title.
[DNLM: 1. Endocrine System Diseases—therapy. 2. Complementary
Therapies—methods. 3. Endocrine Glands—physiopathology. WK
140 B367i 2009]
RC649.B38 2009
616.4'06—dc22   2009014391

ISBN10: 0–7890–3705–X (hbk)
ISBN10: 0–7890–3706–8 (pbk)
ISBN10: 0–203–86913–3 (ebk)

ISBN13: 978–0–7890–3705–3 (hbk)
ISBN13: 978–0–7890–3706–0 (pbk)
ISBN13: 978–0–203–86913–0 (ebk)

To my patients, who have taught me everything.

Contents

List of Illustrations

Figures

Tables

Foreword

Autumn is a spectacular time of the year in Northwest Montana. The crisp temperatures and warm sunlight highlight my favorite season's beautiful foliage. Fall also brings with it cool, damp weather and unstable weather patterns. This is a miserable combination for anyone with rheumatoid arthritis.

In 2002, my life was devastated by rheumatoid arthritis. Every joint in my body was inflamed, I could barely walk, and I was completely exhausted. My livelihood as a chiropractor had depended on health and strength; both were gone. The RA came on insidiously. First this hurt, then that. Then, I could no longer get up in the morning and exercise. I put on two dress sizes for no reason. I was becoming more and more tired. Then one morning I woke up and I could barely walk.

I consulted a rheumatologist who confirmed my greatest health fear. I grew up watching my greataunt "live" with RA. The pain and dysfunction of the disease left her wheelchair bound and imprisoned in nursing homes for over twenty years. In the 1970s and 1980s, RA was treated with medications. Aunt Ida took them all, including gold shots, with no benefit. Her suffering continued until her death. The diagnosis of RA left me feeling hopeless and depressed. I was prescribed medications and physical therapy. I asked my rheumatologist, "If I take these medications, when will it go away?" She told me it would not go away and that I would have it forever. I wasn't even forty years old.

I immediately made an appointment with Dr. Donald Beans. I had already been seeing him for strange symptoms. I realize now these strange symptoms were the slow onset of disease.

Dr. Beans was armed with research. He helped me understand the physiology of the disease. He taught me about the endocrine glands that are affected by the inflammatory process associated with RA. He answered all of my questions. He affirmed my decision to not use prescription medication. I acted on his advice. In doing so, one truth led to another. Within three years the RA was handled! Thank you, Don.

The wisdom in this book is vital for humanity. I see it as a beacon of light for the sick, and a powerful tool for healers.

Michele Larsen D.C.

Acknowledgments

The great minds of natural medicine and of historical endocrinology have illuminated my thinking: Dr. Sajous, one of the first endocrinologists in America, and Dr. Henry Harrower who started the first endocrine clinic in America in Glendale, California in 1922, pointed the way. In addition, special thanks to Harrower's wife Olive, who showed me a personal portrait of the man. Thanks go to Dr. Royal Lee who knew the true nature of holistic medicine and created the Standard Process Company so we can all benefit from his knowledge and wisdom.

I must thank my mentors, Mary D. McFarland for expert guidance in homeopathy and Vasil P. Czorny MD and King Lee for teaching me acupuncture at the highest levels. Dr. Bernard Jensen gave me many opportunities for studying and teaching iridology and nutrition.

Ethan Russo MD believed in the project from the very beginning. Heidi Sue Adams, medical librarian of Kalispell Regional Medical Center was indispensable at the beginning of this project, and was able to find anything requested.

Thanks also to my long-suffering friends and relatives who have endured the many discussions of writing and of endocrinology, probably beyond the limits.

Also, thanks to honorary Integrative Endocrinologist Ron Brevik who has listened to every detail of this practice along with our mutual friend, Arturo Fuente.

A very special thanks goes to the crew at the Bridge Medical Center, Whitefish Montana. Steven Gordon ND, Patricia Cole MD, Ryan Wigness DC, and our other colleagues have put the true meaning of integrative medicine into practice. A spirit of true cooperation is evident to all who cross our threshold.

I thank my wife Leslie, who has been my constant companion, cheerleader and mentor on this adventure of a first book.

A very special thanks to the people who provided the figures, adding so much to this text.

For the Spectro-Chrome drawings, Figures 9.1 and 9.2, Darius Dinshah.

For the foot reflexology chart, Figure 12.1, Kevin and Barbara Kunz.

For the excellent iris charts, Figures 12.2 and 12.3, Art Jensen, the son of my friend and teaching associate Dr. Bernard Jensen.

For the chart of the location of the endocrine glands on page 67 of this book, Diane Ableoff, her expertise is neurosurgical textbooks.

For the feedback loops in endocrinology on page 68 of this book, Williams Textbook of Endocrinology (2003) 10th ed., Philadelphia, PA: W.B. Saunders.

Dr. Frank J. Nordt, of Rhein Consulting Laboratories, for the "Twenty-four Hour Urine Hormone Profile" drawings in the Appendix to this book.

1 Introduction

Integrative Endocrinology: The Rhythms of Life is the first book to describe and teach the practice of using multiple natural therapies to treat the endocrine system. Integrative endocrinology is the combined use of Western bedside diagnosis, clinical laboratory examination, and Oriental and other complimentary and alternative medical methods to assess the function of the endocrine system, and treat early endocrine disorders by natural healing methods.

Divisions of the text are as follows: a history and philosophy section, including a brief introduction to each of the natural therapies, and a diagnosis and treatment section organized under a heading for each endocrine gland. This text teaches clear diagnostic criteria and exacting treatment protocols for each endocrine gland and each treatment method.

This book serves the practitioner looking for basic endocrine information and a wide variety of natural treatment options in one text. In addition, the motivated layperson seeking to understand the complexities of the endocrine system, without having to decipher a host of medical textbooks, will benefit.

Since time immemorial, man has recognized a normal pattern to the health of individuals and the many deviations from that normal state. Various points of view proposed many explanations for these diseases: medical, spiritual, philosophical, and cultural.

Oriental medical practitioners use either the Law of Five Elements or the Differentiation of Syndromes. The Ayurvedic physicians of India use three energy parameters or Doshas, namely Vatta, Pitta, and Kapha. A dynamic balance of the three Doshas equals health. Hippocrates (460–370 BC) used the theory of the humors. Early writings suggest an indefinite number, but four humors, blood, phlegm, black bile and yellow bile, became core in the work of Galen.

Galen (131–201 AD) sought to codify and unify all Western medical thinking before him. Medicine used Galen's codified form of practice for 1400 years, a measure of his success.

Similia similibus curentur—"Let likes be treated by likes"—is a medical truism used by Hippocrates and Paracelsus (1493–1541), but never as completely as by Hahnemann (1755–1843). Hahnemann, the originator of homeopathy, taught that all healing must proceed using the law of similars. He added to the idea of similars the pharmaceutical technique of succusion and serial dilution, thereby removing any adverse effects of a medicine and increasing its dynamic potential.

Many of the ancient Chinese remedies are "similars," for example, using liver from an animal to treat a human liver disorder. Sun Su Mo elucidated this treatment strategy in his text *Chen Chin Fang* (*The Thousand Golden Prescriptions, c.* 618 AD).

The use of similars was also the basis for glandular feeding used in early endocrinology and the reasoning behind Brown–Sequard's self-injections, leading to the beginning of modern endocrinology.

Based on these philosophical frameworks and others, practitioners created and developed various types of medicinals to return the ill person to health. *Medicinals* is the term used throughout the text to mean any substance taken into the body to effect a positive change in health. These substances can originate from plants (herbs), minerals, or animal life, such as gland cell extracts.

Longevity proves the success of these methods. For hundreds or even thousands of years, some of these methods have been used to treat human ailments.

Hormone replacement therapy (HRT) supplanted many of the useful treatments of early endocrinology. HRT involves the use of hormones pharmaceutically produced and given as a substitute to replace the function of an endocrine gland. The use of hormones is very attractive to physicians and patients because it offers instant relief of symptoms. However, taking hormones has no healing or building effect on the endocrine gland. Hormone replacement therapy substitutes for the action of the gland. An integrative approach allows immediate symptom relief, using therapies like acupuncture or herbs, and long-term healing and even rebuilding the gland through proper nutrition and using glandular extracts or herbs.

As has been true in times past and across cultures, many people believe that the knowledge currently held is the ultimate truth. This bias was present when Pliny the Elder completed his *Natural History* in about 72 AD. This bias is still visible in current medical texts. All the time-honored medical systems mentioned include useful truths that current medical thinking should not completely discard.

In the West, especially in the United States, we think of our medical system as the best and firmly based on scientific and rational principles. This is a myth, that is, a belief system without substantiation. In fact, the Office of Technology Assessment reviewed current medical practice in the United States to determine how much day-to-day practice was tested by the scientific method. Its 1978 report, *Assessing the Efficacy and Safety of Medical Technologies*, astonished those who believe in the myth of modern scientific medicine. The authors concluded "only 10 to 20 percent of all procedures currently used in medical practice have been shown to be efficacious by controlled trial."

Pioneering endocrinologist Dr. Henry Harrower was fond of quoting Crile and saying that a useful therapy must pass the test of the "crucible of the clinic." This is the real test of any kind of medicine.

Critics of some therapies advocated in this book object that they are unproven by current medical testing standards and, therefore, should not be considered useful medical interventions. Rather than worry about whether a therapeutic intervention will stand up to a double blind, placebo crossover trial, why not look at its venerable history of successfully treating many patients over the course of many years?

Many modern medicines are tested by double blind, placebo crossover trial, and only after being released into general use are their true side effects brought to light.

In fact, many of the therapies in this text have been subjected to clinical trials and repeatedly been shown to be effective. Many of these studies, conducted by the National Institutes of Health and major universities, are not common knowledge.

In actual practice, it might be better to use the "double conscious" research model developed by Dr. Gordon Alles. In this method, the practitioner understands the value of the therapy and shares this with the patient. In this way, the therapy and the consciousness of the practitioner and patient are brought to bear on the problem at hand. Using this method, we as a society could see the real capabilities of our therapies and medicines.

Despite seeming advances in medical technology, the incidence of many chronic and degenerative diseases is on the rise. The use of drugs and surgery as the main therapeutic tools of ordinary medicine is not addressing many common problems. In the realm of endocrinology, the American medical system has completely adopted the use of hormone administration—oral, injectable, or by the transdermal route—as a substitute for the function of the glands.

This can even go so far, as in some thyroid disorders, that the gland is purposely destroyed in order for it to be replaced by the lifelong prescription of a synthetic hormone.

Certainly, if an endocrine gland completely fails, the use of a synthetic hormone—whether true synthetic, recombinant, or bioidentical—may be the only choice available for sustaining life. This is true in some forms of diabetes where the choice is insulin, or degeneration and death.

As the choice to replace endogenous hormones with synthetic substances receives scientific scrutiny, more problems than solutions seem to be emerging. Unrecognized until studied, the problems must have existed before.

Synthetic hormone replacement for menopausal women, in use for many years, when finally studied showed "the incidence of breast cancer, all histologic types combined was increased by 60–85% in recent long-term users of Hormone Replacement Therapy" (Chen *et al.*, 2002). In another study, conventional hormone replacement therapy (HRT) was shown to double the risk of dementia. The study followed 4,500 women, aged 65 years and older for an average of 4 years (Shumaker *et al.*, 2003).

The use of an exogenous hormone is the creation of a pharmacological effect, not a nutritive, healing, or rebuilding effect. It is more appropriate to reeducate the patient's own gland to produce the hormone, rather than giving the patient a hormone as a pharmaceutical preparation that has no permanent healing effect.

Hormone use also creates potential glandular involution or atrophy. Discontinuing the hormone can cause a profound upset in the feedback mechanisms of the endocrine system, and there is the possibility of a withdrawal syndrome (Hochberg *et al.*, 2003).

The aftermath of prednisone administration is a good example of glandular involution. After discontinuing prednisone therapy, it is necessary to follow the patient for 1 year because the adrenal gland has not had a chance to fully recover its ability to respond to stress situations as a direct consequence of the suppression of its function by the administration of prednisone. This stress can include surgery, an accident, a severe illness, or mental/emotional stress. If the patient experiences any stress, prednisone therapy must be started again.

Some endocrine glands produce a number of hormones. Science knows only some of these hormones. The presence of endocrine-like effects without a known hormone to stimulate these effects indicates the possibility of other hormones not yet identified. If the practitioner selects only one hormone for therapeutic administration and glandular involution occurs, as with the administration of prednisone, what becomes of the other hormones produced by the suppressed gland? When the bloodstream is flooded with prednisone at many times the physiologic replacement amount, this fills all the receptor sites for cortisol with the synthetic hormone. The pituitary then stops producing adrenocorticotropic hormone (ACTH) because it senses the overabundance of prednisone.

This type of therapy produces many side effects. Some of the side effects are a direct consequence of the high level of prednisone and some are the effects of the involuted adrenal gland not producing other hormones. Prednisone therapy suppresses the production of dehydroepiandrosterone (DHEA), even at relatively low doses.

This form of therapy creates a significant change in the hypothalamus–pituitary–adrenal (HPA) axis. Using integrative endocrinology in these cases, the practitioner must consider the effect on all three glands of the HPA axis, not just the adrenals.

There is a related effect when administrating a single high-potency nutrient without the cofactors necessary for that nutrient to function in the body. Either the nutrient is excreted unused, or more often, a depletion of the cofactors is created, leading to a drug-like side effect.

This potential for the creation of a side effect has been clearly shown in new research on vitamin E. Researcher Kenneth Hensley has shown that alpha tocopherol, the most popular form of vitamin E supplement sold in stores, once thought to be the main cardioprotective and anticarcinogenic form of vitamin E, taken at the usually prescribed dose, causes a depletion in gamma tocopherol. The depletion of gamma tocopherol leads to a decrease in the cardioprotective results expected with vitamin E (Hensley, 2004).

You must consider another factor when using high-potency vitamins and minerals or hormones: the chemical (hormone or nutrient) may also block a receptor site.

Because of blockage, the receptor site is no longer available. Blocking of a receptor site is the action of xenoendocrines. This can happen with prescription hormones for female hormone replacement therapy for the symptoms of menopause or as a side effect from plastics or petrochemicals present in food or absorbed from a polluted environment.

This is similar to the use of synthetic vitamins that have a definite effect in the body but are pharmacological, not nutritive. There are similar deleterious effects with prescribed hormones, recommended supplements in a chemical and high-potency form, and xenoendocrines from the environment. All three of these chemically based substances expose the body to unnaturally high doses of powerful elements. These elements are very likely to cause side effects not related to their intended purpose.

Another way to examine the problem of using high potency, synthetic vitamins is to explore vitamin C content in the body. The adrenal gland is the tissue in the body that contains the highest amount of vitamin C (4.5 mg per gm of gland weight). This equals less than 50 mg in both adrenal glands. A typical dose of synthetically produced vitamin C is 1 to 5 gm per day. Compare that amount to the level of vitamin C in the adrenal tissue. What effect is this vitamin C dose having in the body? Is that much necessary or even useful? To be more compatible with human physiology, why not give foods or supplements made from foods that contain naturally occurring amounts of nutrients?

Another problem with synthetically produced vitamins is their origin. At present, 90 percent of the vitamin C produced for the world comes from Chinese pharmaceutical manufacturers. This means that the vitamin C pills you buy in the health food store are almost certainly from this source.

This text recommends taking foods or supplements that are, as a whole, as raw and natural as is possible. The best supplements are those that are as close as possible to the way the substance occurs in nature. One example is the use of glandular material derived from animals. Many manufacturers freeze dry or dehydrate their products. These substances do work; however, the superior method is desiccation that involves drying by use of a vacuum chamber at room temperature. Desiccation preserves as many vitamins and enzymes as possible, with current technology. The application of heat or cold during processing of glandular substances can adversely affect their quality.

Understanding the work of Dr. Royal Lee (1885–1967) makes it possible to fully comprehend the reasons for recommending only whole food vitamin complexes and herbs instead of synthetically produced vitamins or standardized herbs. Royal Lee was a dentist, food pioneer, and founder of the Standard Process Company. In his lectures, Dr. Lee liked to ask which part of a watch makes it possible to tell the time (Lee, 2004). Of course, it is the whole watch, not any one part, and the synergistic interaction between the many parts that enable the telling of time. Taking out one part, the watch could no longer function as a timepiece. Although all the components could still be present, if they were not functioning synergistically, the watch would not function properly.

Apply this metaphor to the use of nutrients. Remove any part of a vitamin complex as it occurs in nature (i.e., food), and the vitamin complex cannot have its intended nutritive effect in the body.

The same inability to properly function in the body is true of a standardized herb. The process of standardization adds a specific amount of the ingredient supposedly responsible for medicinal action to a certain quantity of whole, raw material. This process changes the balance of chemical elements that were originally in the herb as it occurs in nature. Using this process unnaturally changes the balance of micronutrients that require the presence of each other to have an effect on the human body. The process of removing an active ingredient to produce a concentrated product is the practice of Western pharmacology.

Dr. Lee asks a second useful question, but does not elaborate. Why doesn't water burn? The answer seems obvious, but with some reflection, it goes to the heart of the difference between natural and synthetic substances. This statement can also help us to see how the parts are not the same as the whole. It is also an excellent example to explore the concepts of synergy and dissolution.

A molecule of water (H_2O) contains two atoms of hydrogen and one atom of oxygen. Combining the three atoms in this way, they have very specific qualities unique to water, especially when used as a nutrient in the human body. However, by subjecting water to a small amount of electricity, electrolysis takes place. This breaks the water into its component parts.

Mixing these two gases and exposing them to a flame, makes them very flammable, even explosive. The actions of the components of a simple compound such as water bear little resemblance to the original compound.

This is equally true of vitamins, minerals, foods, and herbs. Researchers and doctors go to great lengths to describe the difference between natural progesterone and its synthetic analogs. Dr. John Lee points out that, with only one molecule difference, the progesterone is no longer bioidentical and does not have the same function as its natural counterpart produced in the body (Lee, John 1999). Dr. John Lee then recommends vitamin C, meaning ascorbic acid as sold in any store, which is identical to a vitamin C complex found in food. Doing this, the doctor assumes the same effect in the body of both the natural and synthetic vitamin C.

Dr. John Lee, and many others, apparently do not realize that one synthetic (progesterone) with an incorrect or nonnatural effect in the body is the same as another (vitamin C as ascorbic acid). He prescribes a bioidentical hormone and a synthetic vitamin. These vitamins are synthetic, something a plant or animal never produced and something no human should eat.

In practice, we must remain conscious of these innate biases in our education. Prescribing natural substances has a healing, building, and nutritive effect in the body. Prescribing synthetic substances has a pharmacological effect. One purpose of this text is to help the practitioner recognize the difference between natural and synthetic and provide patients with this information, so they may heal.

The purpose of using the various physical techniques in this book is to reestablish nerve flow, blood flow, or, as in the case of acupuncture, the flow of intrinsic energy or Qi (chi) to the endocrine gland.

Long before the absolute failure of a gland, signs and symptoms of dysfunction present themselves to the trained eye. The previously mentioned medical systems as well as many others offer clues to the change in the functioning of the human body. The therapeutic methods outlined in this book offer time-tested medical approaches to treat disharmonies and return the body to functional or even structural integrity.

Integrative endocrinology will help the practitioner go beyond the recommendations of one system and use combined approaches from many medical systems, in the patient's best interest. Much of the information presented in this text is from traditional, even ancient, sources. Many of these forms of medicine relied solely on the skill of observation and palpation by the practitioner. In Western medicine, this is termed *bedside diagnosis*. Clinical science now gives practitioners the potential to use laboratory tests for the evaluation of endocrine function, but many practitioners rely on lab values too much. Assuming the accuracy of lab values can be a mistake: values received from one lab often do not give the same clinical picture as those from another.

Also, lab values may not match the patient's clinical symptom picture. Hence, strict reliance on these tests is not advisable. In "The Endocrine Patient" Dr. Daniel D. Federman points out, "It is easy to be seduced by numbers and to consider the laboratory report the final arbiter. In fact, it is the history and physical examination, plus the clinician's judgment, that establish the prior probability of a given diagnosis... The clinician's judgment is still the key component of the [diagnostic] process" (Federman, 2003).

Laboratory values viewed without clinical judgment and an appropriate history and physical examination tell us little about the patient's health. Integration of the patient's history and symptoms, the practitioner's observation of signs, and laboratory data will give the clearest and most useful clinical picture on which to base diagnosis and therapy.

The wide variety of techniques presented in *Integrative Endocrinology: The Rhythms of Life* allows the practitioner a great deal of latitude in treatment options. Many of the included techniques are available to any practitioner, that is, homeopathy, herbs, or food supplements. Some specialized methods, like chiropractic and acupuncture, can only be used by licensed practitioners. However, by learning more about the use of these methods to treat glandular disorders, practitioners can make beneficial referrals.

The underlying philosophical point is that many modalities of healing have considered the endocrine glands and developed diverse treatment protocols for healing the endocrines in very specific ways. The core of integrative endocrinology is to look at the treatment of early endocrine disorders as if examining a jewel of many facets. Each facet contributes, in its own way, to the brilliance of the entire gem. In the same way, each treatment modality adds to the complete treatment of the endocrine disorder. Each treatment modality can contribute, in its way, to the enhancement of endocrine function. Some patients will respond to one therapy and other patients will require a different therapy or combination of therapies to accomplish healing.

Use this book as a hologram. Each part interrelates to every other part of the book. The acupuncture chapter must be integrated with the adrenal chapter and the hypothalamus and pituitary chapters as well as the color and herb chapter, and so on, in order to best formulate a diagnosis and an integrated treatment protocol for each individual. Just as there are intimate feedback mechanisms in the endocrine system that create the cohesive functioning of the entire system, so there are interrelations in integrative endocrinology that will help the practitioner see the whole case and understand the individual patient.

Initially, support of the function of the glandular system and other related tissues is paramount. The ultimate aim, however, is rebuilding the gland or tissue, if possible, so it may return to its normal function without the continued use of supplementation or therapy. The goal of integrative endocrinology is to return patients to a healthy state and keep them there.

The healthy state is determined by a patient's genetic inheritance, the penetrance of those genetic tendencies, and the patient's life circumstances. Shakespeare wrote, "Everything that lives must die, passing through nature to eternity" (Shakespeare, 1601). By using the natural methods outlined in this text, the passage may be made more effortlessly and with greater and more harmonious functioning than might otherwise be possible.

Introduction to Therapy Chapters

In this section, we will examine a number of natural (nonpharmaceutical, nonsurgical) therapies that have shown effectiveness in treating the endocrine glands and their related disorders. These chapters are not a complete introduction to each of these therapies; rather, they are for the practitioner who wants a brief introduction to each of these modalities. After reading this section, you will have a general knowledge of each therapy. This knowledge will be enough to start using these methods to benefit your patients and as a starting point for more extensive research into some of the individual practices. To aid in further study, use the texts in the Reading List. These texts are a good start on a library of reference for integrative endocrinology.

Each therapy is presented with some history and information about its practical application in the clinic or as a therapy administered to the patient at home. In addition to the general information, there are gems of practical experience that are hard to find elsewhere.

It is the author's hope that you and your patients will use these therapies in the appropriate combination in your clinical setting to benefit the patient's endocrine health in a completely natural way.

2 Acupuncture

Acupuncture is one of the oldest forms of medical practice in the world. When the *Huang Di Nei Jing* (*Yellow Emperor's Classic of Internal Medicine*) was compiled between 500–300 BC, it was a complete work on Chinese medicine, and it is still a useful reference today. The Yellow Emperor, credited with the information in the book, lived in China around 2674 BC. A book compiled so long ago explains the different types of needles and the techniques for their use, information still accurate today.

This is in stark contrast to many other medical systems that have changed their theoretical foundations and practice methods many times in the same historical period. The *Nei Jing* also codifies a complete system of Oriental diagnosis and therapeutic principles. Thousands of books exist explaining Chinese medicine, but the *Nei Jing* clearly shows the longevity and continuity of the practice.

Acupuncture is practiced in countries outside China, especially in the Orient. Japan, Korea, Vietnam have developed their own styles of practice, as have France, Germany, and England. The basic tenets, however, are consistent. In the West, acupuncture was not well accepted until recently. "One is struck by the very varying lapses of time between the original observations of Europeans in China and their publication in the west, as also by their extreme incompleteness, so that it would be fair to say that the full systematization of the Chinese acu-tracts (meridians) and acu-points was never appreciated by westerners until our own time" (Needham, 1980).

Now acupuncture is accepted in nearly every country in the world, with regulation and licensure in many. Books on acupuncture are published in nearly every language.

The first information to appear in a book in the West was *Historia Naturalis et Medica Indiae Orientalis* in 1658 by Dane Jacob de Bondt. However, de Bondt paid no attention to the system of energy flow in the meridians or the relationship of pulse diagnosis to needling technique. Because of the incomplete information provided by de Bondt and other authors, Western countries developed a misunderstanding of the real energetic nature of acupuncture. Now, with a number of schools in the United States and many volumes of Chinese medicine both newly written and English translations of Chinese texts, a full appreciation of diagnosis and treatment is available in the West.

There are many explanations of how acupuncture works. These explanations are scattered throughout the text. Here is one of this author's theories based on Einstein's work. Albert Einstein won the Nobel Prize in 1921 for his explanation of the photoelectric effect. The core of his explanation was that light occurred as quanta or photons. When light shines onto metal, the input of the photons of light causes a measurable output of electrons from the metal. Increasing the frequency of the light but not the intensity can increase the output of electrons from the metal. Chinese acupuncture needles are made with a steel shaft and a copper wound handle that is electroplated with silver. This needle, when inserted into the body, contacts the sodium and potassium ions in the fluid of the body tissues. The author believes that the microcurrent initiated by the needle insertion and activating the depolarization and repolarization of the cell membranes by sodium and potassium could be the reason for the acupuncture effect.

Acupuncture therapy is accomplished by the stimulation of specific points on the body. A separate acupuncture system concentrates on stimulating points located on the ear. The purpose of this stimulation, whether on body or ear points, is to affect the movement of Qi (chi)—the intrinsic energy of life—as it courses through the body along pathways called meridians. In Oriental medical theory, Qi affects every body process including thoughts and feelings. To be in a state of health, a person's Qi must move smoothly along its course, unimpeded by physical injury, poor dietary habits, a disease process, or emotional stress.

Assessing the movement of a person's Qi is necessary to select the appropriate acupuncture points. These points, when stimulated, will return the Qi to a smooth flow, returning the person to a state of health. The meridian system through which Qi flows consists of twelve organ meridians and eight extraordinary vessels. The twelve organ meridians, although they each have different names and pathways, are not separate entities as they might appear to be on an acupuncture chart. The meridians are twelve parts of one continuous flow of energy that circulates throughout the human body. The eight extraordinary vessels are ancillary pathways for the movement of Qi connected to the twelve organ meridians.

Supporting diagnosis in Oriental medicine are the "Two Pillars," the pulse and the tongue. Assessing the movement of Qi by observation of the tongue is a very direct matter. Certain areas of the tongue correspond to specific acupuncture meridians.

Observe the shape of the body of the tongue, its color, and its coat. This information and a look at the chart of correspondences is all that is needed. With practice, a very quick look at the patient's protruded tongue provides a whole body energy analysis. If the body of the tongue is bright red, this indicates too much heat or an excess of energy in the corresponding meridian. If the tongue's color is dark red or purple, then the area is congested or the blood in that area is stagnant. Tongue diagnosis takes a little practice. Many books show photographs of different tongue presentations and their accompanying diagnoses.

The use of the pulse in Oriental medicine differs greatly from the use of the pulse in the West. Pulse diagnosis is a system of palpation of twelve separate and distinct pulses on the radial artery at the wrist. The specific quality and amplitude of each pulse is a direct reflection of the energy flowing in the meridian or energy conduit that relates to that pulse. Books on pulse taking can be very useful in honing this invaluable diagnostic skill, but to learn Oriental pulse diagnosis, there is no substitute for an experienced teacher.

The highest ideal of acupuncture treatment is to harmonize the meridian energies reflected in the pulse and the tongue to a state of dynamic equanimity. This is the domain of a person fully trained in acupuncture and Oriental medicine. There are, however, many ways of using the acupuncture system to help specific endocrine disorders, even to the point of teaching the patient a few case-specific acupuncture points for use at home.

The Chinese name for acupuncture is *jinjiu*, meaning needle/heat. The heat refers to moxabustion. Moxa is made from the herb *Artemisia vulgaris*. The leaves of the plant are dried and ground into a coarse powder. The practitioner uses the dried herb in several ways to stimulate the acupuncture points. Burning a small quantity of moxa on the handle of an acupuncture needle while it is in place in the acupoint is one method. Another way to use moxa is to place a small cone on a thin slice of ginger or onion laid on the acupoint. The small cone of moxa is then set alight. The herb does not burn with a flame but smolders until it is burned away, leaving a small amount of ash. In addition, moxa is burned directly on the skin as a small piece made the size of a grain of rice. Burning moxa directly on the skin is a tricky technique. To master this technique, some direct instruction is necessary.

Moxa sticks are also available. The moxa stick is the size and shape of a cigar, set alight and held near the point to create a warm sensation. When the patient feels the sensation change from warm to hot, move the moxa to another point and repeat the process. When all the points selected for that patient have been heated three times, this is considered a treatment. Repeating this process daily in difficult cases is acceptable. The moxa stick is a perfect technique to send home with the patient. There is no need to be exacting in point location as with a needle.

The term acupuncture is a misnomer and reflects a misperception by Jesuit priests in China. They saw only the needle—"acu" in Latin—puncturing the skin, ignoring the heat that is often used.

There are many specialized acupuncture techniques. A specialized use of acupuncture does not take into account the traditional method of diagnosis through the pulse and tongue and other Oriental diagnostic procedures. These diagnostic processes allow the practitioner to arrive at a holistic energetic diagnosis and then perform acupuncture treatment to harmonize the person's entire energy system. This method is truly holistic and ultimately returns the person to a state of health.

Acupuncture treatment to relieve a painful condition is an example of specialized use. Even many years ago, this style was known in the United States. As an example, the Merck Manual (Merck & Co., 1934) lists these instructions for back pain:

> Acupuncture: Sterilize skin over affected muscle with tincture of iodine and alcohol. Insert 4 or 5 sterile needles (hypodermic needles; bonnet pins) into the muscle at the tender points at right angles to the body surface to a depth of $\frac{3}{4}$ to 1 inch. Leave them in place for 5 to 10 minutes.

Although called acupuncture, this technique is more like Janet Travell's "Trigger Point Therapy" (Travell, 1983).

Pain-control acupuncture therapy is quite common. The purpose of treatment is a single focus of pain or pathology and not on the holistic well-being of the patient. Medical practitioners whose training is not primarily Oriental use this acupuncture style for symptomatic relief. This style uses acupuncture as a therapy or an adjunctive technique rather than a complete medical approach.

Describing the location of acupuncture points in ancient times was vague at best. For example, a translation of two of the *Ma Dan Yang* 12-star acupoints from the *Great Compendium of Acupuncture* are as follows: The 36th point on the stomach meridian (St-36; *Zu San Li*) is described as "San Li 3 cun below eye of the knee between the two sinews." The fifth point on the heart meridian (H-5; *Tong Li*) is "Tong Li, Side and behind the wrist, from the wrist 1 cun" (Yang JiZhou, 1981). The writing seems to function only as a memory device for those who learned by example in a traditional teacher–student apprenticeship format.

Over time, the locations were described in increasingly precise terms, leading to the idea that the points have a permanently fixed location. Here is an example of the descriptions of the same two points from a modern text: "Location: St-36, below the knee, 3 cun inferior to St-35, one finger breadth lateral to the anterior crest of the tibia." "Location: H-5, on the radial side of the tendon flexor carpi ulnaris, 1 cun proximal to H-7" (Deadman, 2001) .

The locations of the acupoints are as different as the physical characteristics of each person's body type or facial features. They are not in a permanently fixed location, the same in every person.

The point location information in textbooks is designed to bring the practitioner's hand to the approximate location of the point. Once the practitioner's hand is near the point, they must then use skill and knowledge of underlying anatomy, along with the patient's response to pressure and electrical, heat, cold, or other physical characteristics felt by the practitioner's locating finger, to accurately find the point on an individual patient. The location of an acupoint may vary from person to person. The only way to accurately find acupoints is to practice. Similarly, a surgeon or anatomist will say that anatomical structures do not have a precise location. Anatomical texts are sketches, not blueprints. They show an average or an approximation of location, not a fixed and immovable location.

A Chinese axiom says it takes 3 years of continuous practice to become proficient in the use of acupuncture. In using acupuncture for work in integrative endocrinology, either in a clinical setting or as a self-help technique for patients, familiarity with the point locations is essential. Continuous practice is the only way to achieve this goal. The descriptions of acupoints in this text will be in the modern style. Using pressure, heat, or electrical stimulation, the location is much less critical than with a needle.

If there is a dysfunction of the gland relating to a particular acupoint, the point may exhibit to the patient or the practitioner some difference from the surrounding tissue. The point may be hotter, colder, swollen, more or less painful, discolored, or even totally lack sensation.

Various methods can test the reactivity of a point or meridian. These point-location techniques include palpation, the use of various electrical devices, or the Japanese technique of Akabani. Investigation of the these techniques will allow the use of more acupoints than just the specific points mentioned in each gland chapter.

Another reason for using one of the previously mentioned reactivity testing methods is selecting from among the glandular points for the individual patient, instead of using every point mentioned for a particular gland.

Using palpation, look for the previously mentioned changes in texture, temperature, color, or sensation.

The use of electrical devices creates a tendency to rely on the reading of the electrical meter as if it were precisely reliable. These measurement devices are only as accurate as the operator is. Meters range in price from $200 to $20,000. All these devices operate in essentially the same way. They measure the resistance or the conductivity between a selected acupuncture point and the ground wire held by the patient. If the resistance is high, that is, a low meter reading, the acupuncture meridian and the selected point being tested are said to be blocked or congested and in need of treatment to unblock the point and its associated meridian. If the conductivity is high, that is, a high meter reading, then the meridian and point are overactive or inflamed and need a sedation treatment. The problem with strict reliance on the meter reading is that so many things not related to the acupuncture point or meridian can dramatically affect the reading and, therefore, the diagnosis. If the skin is too moist or too dry, this can adversely affect the reading. Skin moisture increases the conductivity, giving an unusually high reading. The opposite is true for dry skin. The pressure on the stylus used for the measurement can change the reading if not applied the same on each point or each measurement. Imprecise point location will alter the reading.

The other function these machines are said to have is the ability to compare the electrical reading of the acupuncture meridian with the electrical reading of various homeopathic remedies, herbs, or nutritional supplements that have been previously digitally stored in the device. This presents a very complicated problem.

Using sound recording as an analogy helps to explain this difficulty. The original sound recordings done by Edison were strictly mechanically vibrational. As the air movement causing the sound hit the diaphragm of the recording device, it caused the diaphragm to move and caused a needle connected to the diaphragm to move. The moving needle cut a groove in a rotating cylinder, etching the movement of the needle on to the wax.

Reversing the process, the cylinder rotated, to cause the needle to move, creating movement in the diaphragm, which caused the air next to the device to move, recreating the original sound. The process is nearly identical when using an electromagnet instead of the needle or when using magnetic tape. These methods recreate every sound on the recording. This type of recording is an analog recording.

The other type of audio recording is digital. The recording process is similar except that the sound information is stored as binary digits, 1s and 0s, in digital format. Essentially, this process removes all nuances in the recording, eliminating any background noise as well as many musical overtones.

The sounds that are not just the pure musical note contribute to the richness of the analog recording. Digital recording creates a "pure signal." This pure sound is not the same as the sound created by a musical instrument or by the human voice. These natural sounds have many overtones and other vibrations that make them unique. Many music lovers believe that the process of digitizing music destroys many of the qualities of an analog recording.

The same problem exists when the vibration of a homeopathic remedy or a nutritional supplement is digitized for storage and later retrieval. Using the remedy information stored in an electronic device, the device makes a comparison between a synthetic and digitized signal and the vibration created by the meridian or acupuncture point being tested. The digitized signal is not an accurate representation of the original substance and, therefore, not appropriate to use for diagnosis or treatment.

In the late 1970s, the author had the opportunity to study with Dr. Reinhold Voll MD and Dr. Paul Nogier MD, both great proponents of electrical devices for the body and ear acupuncture points, respectively.

Dr. Voll was the originator of EAV (electroacupuncture), according to Dr. Voll, the first real use of electromeasurement devices with acupuncture for medical purposes. Few of Dr. Voll's students or the students of other great teachers produced equally spectacular results as did their teachers.

The careful practitioner must rely on clinical judgment above all else. Then and only then can such instruments be useful. To rely strictly on the measurements of the instrument is bad practice. The instrument is only one tool in the clinical evaluation of the case.

Akabani is a Japanese technique accomplished by holding a joss or incense stick near the terminal acupoint at the end of each meridian, rotating the stick in a small circle over the point until the patient feels a hot sensation. The practitioner notes the number of seconds elapsed before the patient feels the change from warm to hot. By comparing the number of seconds it takes the end point of each meridian to feel hot, the practitioner can judge the relative amount of energy flowing in each meridian. If one meridian endpoint takes 5 seconds to become hot and all the rest take 11 seconds, the 5-second meridian is overactive compared to the others. This means the meridian is unable to accept more energy in the form of heat because it is already carrying too much, relative to the other meridians.

The opposite is true if the meridian endpoint takes a long time to become hot. This method may also be used to introduce heat into a particular acupoint for treating the associated endocrine gland. Teaching this technique to the patient is helpful, so treatment can proceed on a daily or alternating day schedule if the gland is particularly imbalanced.

There is an associated acupuncture point on the ear that accesses every organ in the body. The ear is palpated with an instrument like the blunt end of an acupuncture needle or the insertion tube from a Japanese-style needle or a probe, like a dental tool, which is rounded on the end for this purpose. Many acupuncture supply catalogs offer these devices. A quick assessment can be made of the entire endocrine system as represented in the ear. If the patient feels a sharp or piercing pain then use a gold needle for treatment. The gold needle causes a tonifying effect on the point. If the patient's sensation is dull or spreads out from the point of contact then use a silver needle. The silver needle causes a sedating effect on the point. If the sensation is not defined either way, use a stainless steel needle. The steel needle does not add a tonifying or sedating pressure on the point but allows the body to react to the stimulation in the best way possible (Figure 2.1).

A discovery of Dr. Nogier, the VAS or vascular auricular sign (alternately called vascular autonomic signal) is a technique used for diagnosis in ear

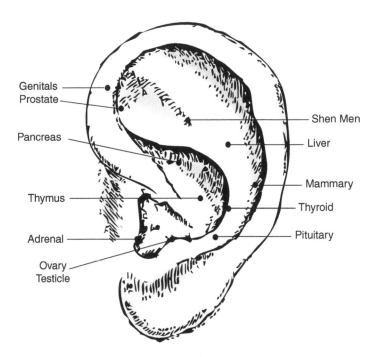

Figure 2.1 Ear Acupuncture Points.

acupuncture. The patient is in the supine position, with the practitioner seated at the head of the table. The practitioner holds the wrist of the patient with the thumb contacting the radial artery at the wrist. The practitioner places the center of the tip of the thumb perpendicularly to the patient's wrist. The exact placement is crucial to get an effective feedback from the patient's body. This placement is half way between the high point of the styloid process of the radial bone and the lowest point. The practitioner may check the correct placement of the thumb by moving the other hand over the patient's arm closely, but without touching it, from the elbow to the wrist, and slowly (approximately 1 to 2 seconds for one pass).

Feel the pulse of the radial artery on the side of the thumb closest to the elbow. Now, reverse the direction of the hand movement from the wrist to the elbow. If the thumb is placed correctly, the pulse of the radial artery is at the distal or hand side of the thumb. It may take some practice to do this successfully. Once mastered, this technique, is essentially muscle testing or applied kinesiology, using the heart reflected through the radial artery. Contacting a point on the ear and feeling the response of the pulse may now assess the need for treatment of any ear point.

When palpating the VAS, use a gold and silver hammer to contact the ear. If a positive VAS is felt with the gold side of the hammer touching the point, then select a gold needle for treatment of that point. If the silver side of the hammer produces a positive response of the VAS to the examiner's thumb, then use a silver needle for the treatment.

Selecting points for sedation or tonification is a very important part of the use of acupuncture technique for integrative endocrinology. In each gland chapter, certain acupoints are listed as tonification or sedation points. This means that the effect of tonifying (that is, increasing the energy in a meridian) or sedating (that is, decreasing the energy in that meridian) is a characteristic of that point.

As an example, if the adrenal gland is shown to be underactive, select the point K-7 in the medial ankle as one of the treatment points. K-7 is the tonification point of the kidney meridian. In Oriental medicine, the kidney meridian controls the adrenal gland. Conversely, if the gland is overactive and requires sedation, use K-1 on the bottom of the foot.

The other methods of tonification and sedation of an acupoint deal with needle manipulation, pressure, temperature, or material used to contact the point. Using a needle for tonification, the needle, once in place in the acupoint, is rotated in a clockwise direction with a thrusting motion. If sedation is called for, a counterclockwise motion is used with a pulling, rather than thrusting, manipulation.

To tonify with manual pressure, use a clockwise circular motion; for sedation, use a counterclockwise direction.

Heat is tonifying and cold is sedating. Therefore, ice held in contact with a point sedates and moxa or an incense stick held near the point tonifies.

Combine any of these techniques for increased effect. For instance, to increase the tonifying effect, place a gold needle in the tonification point and manipulate it in a tonifying manner as mentioned previously. This is a way of combining three tonifying strategies.

Another effective way to use acupuncture theory in treating the endocrine system is to use Magrain pellets. The pellets are inexpensive, effective, and easy to use. These small pellets come with a small piece of tape to hold them in place. Their materials are gold, silver, and steel. Once in place on the point, they can remain there for several days. The pellets are available in many acupuncture supply catalogs.

The above techniques for tonification or sedation can be used with any point on the body or the ear. As an example, select the point B-23 to make as direct contact as possible with the adrenal glands. Depending on the diagnosis, select either a sedating or tonifying strategy. The point B-23 is not inherently for either kind of stimulation. Choose one of the above strategies to activate the point and, therefore, the gland, or propagate a slowing signal through the point to the gland, sedating its function.

Another way to use acupuncture theory in treating endocrine disorders is the "Ah Shi" point. The first mention of the Ah Shi point was in the *Thousand Ducat*

(Golden) Prescriptions in the Tang dynasty (618 AD). "The site of pain was considered to be a legitimate site for acupuncture treatment" (Bensky, 1980).

Ah Shi is translated as "oh, yes" or "that's it," meaning a point of pain when pressure is applied or a point on the surface of the body that the patient notices has a different sensation from the surrounding area. The Ah Shi point may not be a known acupoint or be on a known meridian.

This author believes that acupoints and Ah Shi points both function as a two-way street. Stimulation on the point on the surface of the body can create a reaction at an internal and distant location. This is the ultimate theoretical explanation of how acupuncture works. The opposite is also true. If there is an effect or imbalance in an internal area of the body, the meridian pathways allow for a conduit to the body surface of a referred pain, which can be perceived by the patient or the practitioner. These points can be traditional acupuncture points on the body or on the ear or they may be the Ah Shi points as well. Any acupuncture point can function in this two-way street fashion.

Each gland chapter gives instructions on recommended treatment, including which meridians or individual acupoints are usually associated with that gland. The use of these access points in endocrine treatment is invaluable. This method has been used for thousands of years and on millions of people, with great success.

Using the instructions in this book, a practitioner who is not an acupuncturist will not become qualified merely by internalizing what is discussed in this chapter. However, the use of acupoints and those points mentioned in the chapter on neural therapy can allow any practitioner the most direct access to the various glands from the body's surface. This will greatly increase treatment options and the efficacy of individual treatments.

The use of acupuncture points will also allow the patient to participate with the practitioner by carrying out home treatment of the points determined to be of benefit to his or her individual endocrine situation.

Although acupuncture is a complete medical system and many states license the practice, a qualified health professional can learn a few key points for use in integrative endocrinology to give additional stimulation or sedation to a particular gland.

Also, use acupuncture theory as an adjunct to any other technique being used for endocrine balance. Acupuncture is one of the premiere therapies to select when deciding on a therapeutic regimen for any endocrine disorder. Because there are so many techniques available to the practitioner for the stimulation of these points, use of needle stimulation method by those not fully trained is not recommended. However, adequate stimulation can be accomplished by heat, cold, electricity, or even manual pressure.

3 Homeopathy

Homeopathy—a form of medicinal prescribing—originates in the paradigm of Western medicine. Samuel Hahnemann, a German medical doctor, clearly formulated the philosophy and practice of classical homeopathy (Hahnemann, [1842] 1996). The maxim of homeopathy is the Latin phrase *similia similibus curentur*, which means "let likes be treated by likes."

Hippocrates used this phrase. He not only used the treatment by likes or similars, he also used the treatment by opposites in his medical practice, and allopathy, so termed by Hahnemann, is the second form of treatment using opposites. Allopathy is the way ordinary doctors treat disease today. A doctor might use an antiinflammatory drug to treat inflammation and an antibiotic to treat an infection.

Simple examples of these treatment procedures are the application of heat to a burn (similar) and the application of cold to a burn (opposite).

After Hippocrates, Paracelsus used this idea extensively and further developed similars. But never were similars so eloquently and completely used as done by Hahnemann.

The beginnings of Hahnemann's ideas for homeopathy are evident in an article he published in 1796. Another major work of Hahnemann, *The Organon*, published in 1810, elucidated the entire philosophy of homeopathy and the related details of diagnosis and treatment.

He perceived homeopathy when translating a *materia medica* written by Cullen. He noticed that the symptoms of an overdose of Peruvian bark were the same as the symptoms of malaria that, at the time, was the treatment for malaria.

Hahnemann pondered three important points. First, what is the smallest dose that will display symptoms in a healthy person? Second, what is the smallest dose that could treat malaria? Third, what other substances create symptoms that they also cure?

Through absolute and pure experimentation on humans, he found the answers to these three questions and began treating people with homeopathic remedies. It is interesting to note that this experimentation far predates Claude Bernard (1813–1878) the French physiologist, known as the father of experimental medicine.

Hahnemann used the term *provings* to define the experiments he performed. The following are some of the steps in proving. A group of healthy volunteers were orally administered a homeopathically prepared (explained later), pharmacologically active substance. The members of the experimental group continue to take the substance until they develop symptoms. The individual prover stops oral administration of the substance as soon as symptoms appear. Throughout the entire proving, symptoms are recorded for up to 1 month after the initial dose. The symptoms experienced by the provers create a clinical picture of the effect of the substance on a healthy person.

In a clinical setting, when a patient describes his or her symptoms to the practitioner, it is necessary to match the symptoms described by the patient as closely as possible to the symptoms reported in the provings. A homeopath uses two types of texts to accomplish this goal.

The first text is *Materia Medica*. The *Materia Medica* lists each remedy name in alphabetical order. Within each remedy chapter, the symptoms of that remedy are organized like a review of systems, similar to history taking in ordinary medicine. The book lists symptoms by body system, starting from the head and proceeding down the body, covering every area.

The second main text of homeopathy is the Repertory. The entire book is organized as a review of symptoms starting from the head and listing all systems and tissues of the body. Each symptom contains a list of abbreviations of the remedies known to have treated that symptom in the past or the symptoms as reported in a proving. These symptoms with their associated remedies are called rubrics.

The remedy abbreviations in the Repertory are graded. A "one" or remedy appearing in plain type is least likely to affect the symptom. A "two" or remedy appearing in italic type is more likely to help that particular symptom. A remedy in bold type is a "three" and has a very strong possibility of curing the problem under consideration. In the Repertory, there are very few "fours"; these remedies are in bold and italic type and are strongly known to be curative for the symptom.

Taking a case (recording the symptoms of the patient), you must heed the strength of the patient's symptoms. How spontaneous, clear, or "strange, rare, and peculiar" are the symptoms?

You must be attentive to the strength of each symptom of the patient. The strongest symptoms have the most weight when analyzing the case.

You must also match the greatest number of the patient's symptoms as possible with the description of the remedy to find the similimum or the exact remedy for your patient. This can be a painstaking process, but it achieves extraordinary results.

Making Homeopathic Remedies

Hahnemann found—and any experienced homeopath of today can tell you—that the more preparation steps a substance has gone through, the deeper acting the resulting remedy is.

The substances that are called homeopathic remedies are prepared in the following manner. We will use tincture of Belladonna as an example. A tincture is an alcohol extract, in this case of the deadly nightshade plant.

Beginning with the centessimal dilution system, we add one drop of the tincture of Belladonna to 99 drops of pure ethyl alcohol. This mixture is then succussed 100 times. Succussion is the process of striking the vial containing the Belladonna and alcohol against a hard but resilient surface, like a book. When the product of 1 drop to 99 drops is complete, the result is Belladonna 1c. The Arabic numeral (1) indicates the number of dilution steps. The Roman numeral (c) indicates the number of drops used at each dilution step.

The next step is to take one drop of 1c and mix it with 99 drops of alcohol and succuss 100 times again. This product is termed Belladonna 2c. The process of dilution and succussion continues to produce the medicines commonly used in homeopathic prescribing: 3c, 6c, 12c, 30c, and 200c.

When the dilutions reach 1,000 times, the designations change to m, and 1m equals 1,000 dilution and succussion steps, 10m equals 10,000 steps, and 50m equals 50,000 steps. As we progress up the potency scale, the designations change again to be Roman numerals without Arabic numbers, that is, cm or 100,000 and mm or 1,000,000.

There are two other preparation systems for homeopathic remedies. One is called the decimal system and its remedies are designated as 6x or 12x, with the x standing for mixing the original tincture with 10 drops of alcohol instead of the 100 drops used in the centessimal system. The decimal system comes from Europe years after Hahnemann's death. In some countries, especially Germany, a d may substitute for the x.

The LM system is the third system of preparation of remedies for use in homeopathy. This method was in the sixth or final edition of Hahnemann's work *The Organon* (Hahnemann, [1842] 1996). The LM represents

50,000, which means one drop of original or mother tincture is mixed with 50,000 drops of alcohol. This mixture is then succussed. This first process produces LM1. To produce LM2, take one drop of LM1 and add it to 50,000 drops of alcohol and succuss.

Besides the number of drops used in making a remedy, another difference with LM remedies is that, they are succussed 6 to 12 times before each administration. This mild succussion slightly changes the potency each time the remedy is administered.

Hahnemann felt these remedies produced the same healing effect as his centessimal potencies but were gentler to the body and the mind and emotions.

Now that we have seen how the medicines are made, we now need to ask, how can such dilute medicines actually have an effect toward healing? Hahnemann believed in a dynamic force. This force is responsible for all body processes, even all thoughts and emotions. The author has not read any reference in Hahnamann's writing to knowledge of either Ayurvedic healing or Chinese medicine, but both these systems have a very similar viewpoint. The Orientals call this force or energy Qi (Chinese) or Ki (Japanese), and the East Indians call it Prana.

Hahnemann felt that all symptoms a person had were a reflection of this internal energy to the outside world and that indeed the symptoms were the expression of the illness. Dissipating of the symptoms by a medicine indicates that the dynamic energy is changed and the disease is removed.

He also considered a wide range of sensations, signs, behaviors, proclivities, and preferences to be included under the category of symptoms. Not only was the redness and itch of a rash part of the symptom picture but also whether the rash got better by a hot or cold application. Other important symptoms include whether the patient prefers hot or cold drinks and whether the patient wants fresh air or to stay indoors. Hahnemann felt these all indicated the state of the dynamic force, requiring, therefore, the medicine needed to put the dynamic force back to a state where its flow was unimpeded so that life could proceed without obstacles.

The main tenets of classical homeopathy are as follows:

1. The minimum dose (the smallest amount of medicine that will effect a cure).
2. The single remedy (no mixtures of remedies or polypharmacy).
3. The totality of symptoms (using all the symptoms of the individual to find the appropriate remedy).

In each gland chapter, you will find a number of remedies found in the literature that are helpful for each particular gland. Each chapter shows a selection of the top few remedies, giving some of their symptoms and indicating their usefulness for the gland.

You can use the information in the gland chapter and then combine that with the patient's mental and emotional character to arrive at a very satisfactory remedy to supplement the healing of that gland.

So far, this chapter has only mentioned the classical homeopathy of Hahnemann. There are other systems that use homeopathically prepared substances developed in the years since Hahnemann.

One such system is the use of combination remedies. This is a system of combining remedies that have a similar action or that act on similar problems or tissues in a single vial to be administered as a single medicine. Obviously, this violates Hahnemann's idea of the single remedy. Also, these remedies are not proved in the classical sense. However, these combinations have existed for many years, and a sort of proving has taken place by use in clinical practice.

Over many years, thousands of medical practitioners have used these combinations with success. The combinations function more like ordinary medicine rather than as a homeopathic remedy. This means that combination remedies are prescribed for a disease condition but not on the basis of the total picture of the patient's symptoms. Many countries now produce these remedies for oral administration and for injection. One such remedy is Traumeel® from the Heel® Company. This injectable is an extraordinary antiinflammatory, especially when mixed in equal proportions, with procaine 2 percent. This product is equal to or better than the use of cortisone in situations that call for injection of an antiinflammatory.

If a certain remedy is not available to you, it may be necessary to manufacture it yourself. In fact, Hahnemann recommended each physician make all their remedies. He also recommended that physicians test each medicine on themselves to become familiar with the effect. That might have been possible then, but not now. There are thousands of remedies in use today. However, in some circumstances it may be impossible to get a remedy you want. This situation could arise if you wanted to follow the work of the French homeopaths who use hormones made into homeopathic remedies to treat the glandular production of each hormone directly.

Extrapolating the instructions of O.A. Julian for folliculinum, we can see how to use other homeopathic hormone preparations. His instructions are a low potency 3c be used as an arouser, 7c as a regulator, and 9c as a restrainer (Julian, 1979).

Making remedies in these low potencies is easy, if you have access to the original hormone. A method of preparing remedies called the Korsakoff method (Vithoulkas, 1980) is most useful for the individual practitioner.

To use this method to create your own remedy, start with a clean two-dram glass vial. To this vial, add one drop of the hormone you wish to produce in potency. Next, add 100 drops of ethyl alcohol. Succuss this mixture, by striking the vial against a book or your palm, 100 times. The vial now contains the hormone in the potency 1c. You may now discard the liquid in the vial. The amount remaining on the walls of the vial is estimated to be one drop. Add to this drop of hormone 1c, another 100 drops of alcohol. Succuss the mixture 100 times. The vial now contains hormone 2c. Repeat the above steps to obtain hormone 3c. Now with a vial containing 100 drops of hormone 3c, you can moisten a vial of #35 sucrose pellets with a few drops of the liquid. You only need to put enough liquid in the vial to lightly moisten the pellets. You now have a vial for dispensing to the patient and enough hormone 3c to fill perhaps 50 more prescriptions. If you kept a vial of 2c you could make 100 times as much, and beginning with 1c, you could make 1,000 times. This is true because each drop of 2c will make 100 vials of 3c.

To progress to 7c or 9c, simply follow the above instructions and in a few minutes, you will have any hormone or other medicinal substance made into a perfectly usable homeopathic remedy as well made as by any pharmacy.

You must maintain a clean atmosphere when preparing remedies in this way to avoid any contamination. You must also maintain your focus to ensure that you are producing the right remedy, in the right potency.

Homeopathic Research

Conventional medicine often challenges the science of homeopathy. Part of the reason for this is the high dilutions used to produce the remedies. The fact that, in clinical practice, a more dilute substance has a curative effect in the human body greater than a more concentrated substance seems to contradict the laws of ordinary chemistry. This would be true if homeopathy worked by a chemical effect as is true of drugs used in ordinary medicine. However, the action of homeopathic remedies is a dynamic or energetic effect. The dilution does not decrease the action of the remedy. Succussion increases the remedy's energetic potential when it acts on the human energetic system.

In scientific research, a phenomenon is observed, a hypothesis is proposed, and research proceeds to prove or disprove the hypothesis. When ordinary medicine looks at homeopathy, it is dismissed out of hand because they say homeopathy cannot work if there is no substance left in the medicine. In addition, it is said that there is no research to prove the effect of homeopathic remedies or that the effect of homeopathy is simply a placebo.

Actually, many excellent studies of the effect of homeopathic remedies exist. Some of the homeopathic research was published in peer-reviewed mainstream medical journals, some was funded and published by the National Institutes of Health, and other research was done by the U.S. Department of Defense.

Animals have been successfully treated with homeopathy for nearly as long as humans. Even herd animals have been treated experimentally (Day, 1995). Day did an experiment with dairy cattle. Half of a herd was treated with a homeopathic remedy for mastitis and the other half was not treated. The remedy was placed into the water of the treated half. There was a dramatic difference in the number of cases of mastitis in the treated and untreated cattle. The conditions of the experiment were equal, as the cattle were in the same barn.

Some people think that the placebo effect is the mode of action of homeopathy; however, it is often true that the wrong remedy is chosen for the initial prescription and no effect is noted. When the second or sometimes the third remedy is chosen, and if it is the right remedy for the case, then we see the appropriate healing effect. If the effect was simply placebo, it should work better on the first try instead of the third.

Another fact that speaks for the method of homeopathy is the collective clinical experience of thousands of practitioners whose clinical experience, as a group, covers a period of more than 200 years and who use the same methodology consistently.

Simply claiming there is no research does not make it so. Dana Ullman has written three books outlining the many research studies on homeopathy. In addition, the very scholarly work of Harris Coulter documents much of the research conducted in homeopathy (Coulter, 1973). In 1991, three professors of medicine from the Netherlands, none of them homeopaths, performed a meta-analysis of 25 years of clinical studies using homeopathic medicines and published their results in the *British Medical Journal* (Klenijnen *et al.*, 1991). This meta-analysis covered 107 controlled trials, of which 81 showed that homeopathic medicines were effective, 24 showed they were ineffective, and 2 were inconclusive. The professors concluded, "The amount of positive results came as a surprise to us." Specifically, they found the following:

Thirteen of 19 trials showed successful treatment of respiratory infections.
Six of seven trials showed positive results in treating other infections.
Five of seven trials showed improvement in diseases of the digestive system.
Five of five trials showed successful treatment of hay fever.
Five of seven trials showed faster recovery after abdominal surgery.
Four of six trials promoted healing in treating rheumatological disease.
Eighteen of 20 trials showed benefit in addressing pain or trauma.
Eight of ten trials showed positive results in relieving mental or psychological problems.

Thirteen of 15 trials showed benefit from miscellaneous diagnoses.

Despite the high percentage of studies that provided evidence of success with homeopathic medicine, most of these studies had flaws of some kind. Still, the researchers found 22 high-caliber studies, 15 of which showed that homeopathic medicines were effective. Of further interest, they found that 11 of the best 15 studies showed efficacy of these natural medicines, suggesting that the better designed and performed the studies were, the higher the likelihood that the medicines were found to be effective. Although people unfamiliar with research may be surprised to learn that most of the studies on homeopathy had flaws in one significant way or another, research in conventional medicine during the past 25 years has had a similar percentage of flawed studies too.

With this knowledge, the researchers of the meta-analysis on homeopathy concluded, "The evidence presented in this review would probably be sufficient for establishing homeopathy as a regular treatment for certain indications."

Despite the resistance to change in general and to homeopathy specifically, it is becoming increasingly difficult for physicians and scientists to doubt the benefits that homeopathic medicines offer. Italian hematologist Paolo Bellavite and Italian homeopath Andrea Signorini's *Homeopathy: A Frontier in Medical Science* (1995) is presently the most comprehensive resource of controlled studies on homeopathy. The authors conclude, "The sum of the clinical observations and experimental findings is beginning to prove so extensive and intrinsically consistent that it is no longer possible to dodge the issue by acting as if this body of evidence simply did not exist."

Hahnemann was a great advocate of understanding classic literature and philosophy. He felt this was necessary to be a good homeopathic physician because these works often contained universal truths that medicine lacked. One of the main tenets of homeopathy is individualization of the remedy to fit the patient, not the disease. The following quote from Aristotle could have been written by Hahnemann and goes to the heart of homeopathic philosophy.

> For the physician does not cure man, except in an incidental way, but Callias or Socrates or some other called by some individual name, who happens to be a man. If, then, a man has the theory without the experience, and recognizes the universal but does not know the individual included in this, he will often fail to cure; for it is the individual that is to be cured.
>
> (McKeon, 1941)

Hahnemann discovered in the proving of medicines that people reacted with very different symptoms to the same medicine. He also found it necessary to be attentive to the nuances in recording the symptoms of patients.

By means of these pure and accurate investigations we shall be made aware that all the symptomatology hitherto existing in the ordinary system of medicine was only a very superficial affair, and that nature is wont to disorder man in his health and in all his sensations and functions by disease or medicine in such infinitely various and dissimilar manners, that a single word or a general expression is totally inadequate to describe the morbid sensations and symptoms which are often of such a complex character, if we wish to portray really, truly, and perfectly the alterations in the health we meet with.

(Hahnemann, 1842)

4 Gland Cell Therapy

Using the endocrine glands of animals and other tissues to treat disorders of the same gland or tissue in humans is a practice known from the beginning of written medical history. It is at once the beginning of modern endocrinology and one of the most ancient medical practices.

The earliest writings about this therapy in the Western medical tradition begin with Hippocrates. Later, Pliny the Elder in his monumental work *Natural History* devotes many chapters to the use of animal tissues in the treatment of human ailments. Of particular interest is Book 28, which outlines the drugs obtained from animals; Book 29 is about animals and the history of medicine; and Books 30 and 31 conclude his elucidation of the drugs of human medicine obtained from animals. This text, originally in Latin and completed around 67 AD, is translated into English (Pliny, [72] 1938).

From an Oriental perspective, glandular therapy was first codified in the *Chien Chin Fang* compiled by Sun Su Mo around 618 AD. This text describes the use of animal liver to treat human liver ailments and, long before Murray (1891), the use of goat thyroid for the treatment of goiter.

The birthday of modern endocrinology is June 1, 1889, when the renowned French physiologist Charles-Edouard Brown-Sequard reported on his self-injections of a solution made from the testicles of dogs and guinea pigs. Brown-Sequard wrote in *The Lancet*,

> I have made use, in subcutaneous injections, of a liquid containing a small quantity of water mixed with the three following parts: first, blood of the testicular veins; second, semen; and third, juice extracted from a testicle, crushed immediately after it was taken from a dog or a guinea-pig.
>
> (Brown-Sequard, 1889)

He then injected one cubic centimeter of the filtered mixture. He took 10 injections over 20 days.

At the age of 72 years, he felt his strength had been diminishing for 10 to 12 years to the point where he had to sit down after only 30 minutes work in the laboratory. At the end of the day, he would eat hastily at 6 p.m. and go immediately to bed, exhausted. After the injections, he could work for several hours without becoming tired and in the evening after supper, do laboratory work, or write on difficult subjects. For one week before the trial and one month following the first injection, he tested his limb strength with a dynamometer. The results were that his right forearm flexors before the injections measured 32 to 37 kg, and after the injections measured 39 to 44 kg. Twenty-five years earlier, he could lift 40 to 46 kg.

He also measured urination and defecation; both were very much improved after the injections. He began to run up the stairs, which had been his previous custom.

By July 3, 1889, the effect had diminished. He wondered about autosuggestion, but the fact that the results wore off contradicts this idea. Dr. M. G. Variot of Paris tried the same injections on three old men with similar results. He also gave water injections to two patients without effect. None of Variot's patients was aware of Brown-Sequard's work and was told only that they were receiving fortifying injections. This is a small sample, but is still a placebo-controlled trial. By the end of 1889, only a few months after publication of the *Lancet* article, 12,000 physicians were using Brown-Sequard's method (Brown-Sequard, 1889).

Live Cell Therapy is the injection of glandular material from various animals to aid in the recovery of function of the endocrine glands of humans. The credit for this therapy goes to Dr. Paul Niehans MD of Switzerland in 1930. However, there is essentially no difference between Dr. Neihans' therapy and the injections performed by Brown-Sequard in 1889, except perhaps that later in his career Neihans began using fetal glandular tissue to decrease the potential of an anaphylactic reaction, because the fetal cell surface did not contain the immune response-triggering characteristics of adult animals. Neihans also mentions in his book (Neihans, 1960) that the cells can be frozen at a very low temperature and then dehydrated. Lyophilization is the process of freezing and drying glandular material. This method preserves the cells for at least 1 year. Modern laboratories are now preserving cells that are not dried, but kept in a fluid medium under refrigeration; they can be preserved for several years and still remain viable.

Critics of gland cell therapy have a fundamental flaw in their opposition to this age-old practice. They believe that only the hormone produced by a gland can have an effect in the body.

Hans Selye was an endocrinologist from Toronto. He wrote a textbook on endocrinology and was the first to write about the general adaptation syndrome that is the body's reaction to stress. Selye writes, "on the basis of what we know about the chemical properties of the testis hormone, his [Brown-Sequard] extracts could not possibly have contained sufficient amount to produce any detectable effect" (Selye, 1947).

This kind of thinking pervades modern endocrinology as it relates to oral gland cell therapy or cell injection therapy. It also completely ignores the facts of the experiments and the experience of thousands of physicians, because the information does not happen to fit Selye's idea of how the endocrine gland cell therapy works. He does not quote from his personal experience with cell therapy or any experimental evidence, just his own idea.

Expressing the opposite view was Charles Sajous. Sajous writes, "No one who, as I did, saw Brown-Sequard before and after he had submitted himself to this treatment could stretch his imagination sufficiently to attribute the change in his appearance to auto-suggestion. He literally looked twenty years younger" (Sajous, 1922). Sajous was there as a witness to what happened to Brown-Sequard, unlike Selye who is making up what must have happened. Is this another of many attempts to rewrite the history of medicine?

Since Banting's isolation of insulin in 1921 from pancreatic islet cells, the whole of the ordinary medical profession has been focused on isolating the one factor of each gland that causes the greatest and most expeditious effect. Ordinary endocrinology totally ignores any other cofactors or any possibility of rebuilding the gland rather than just replacing its function with an externally administered hormone.

Because of this thinking, ordinary endocrinology is focused on hormone replacement therapy (HRT), whether insulin for the diabetic, estrogen for the menopausal female, thyroxin for deficient thyroid, or testosterone for hypogonadism.

Harvey Cushing, a famous endocrinologist from the early 1900s and pioneer of pituitary surgical techniques, is often held out as one of the early endocrinologists who stood for scientific and rational medicine. Even Cushing advocates glandular feeding by oral administration or injection:

> It was our experience with a series of experimentally hypophysectomized dogs to find that animals suffering from a known deficit of glandular secretion could be benefited by injection of extracts, by glandular feeding or by implantations of hypophyses from other sources. Other animals in whom "nearly total" removals had been performed could, by glandular administration, be permanently tided over the critical post-operative period in which acute symptoms of glandular insufficiency argued a fatal issue, the remaining fragment of the gland in the meantime undergoing a compensatory hyperplasia until it sufficed for the physiologic needs of the animal, at which time the glandular feeding could be safely discontinued.

> Unquestionably these symptoms can be ameliorated by glandular administration in one form or another. In view of the fact that the malady is a polyglandular one, as has been emphasized, the administration

of extracts of glands other than the one primarily involved—at least of glands such as adrenal and thyroid, which show secondary deficiencies—may be of service. Examples are given in the case reports of patients definitely improved by thyroid feeding, and in the case of a eunuchoid giant with signs of secondary hypo-adrenalism (asthenia, pigmentation and low blood pressure) I have seen marked benefit from adrenal administration.

(Cushing, 1911)

It is obvious from Cushing's experience that to him glandular feeding was for rebuilding the glands and not for replacing their function. He was using pituitary, adrenal, and thyroid glandular extract to improve the hormone-producing abilities of those glands.

Experimentation done in Germany and Austria has produced some interesting results that indicate that it is not the hormone content of glandular administration that is responsible for its action. Schmid makes it clear that the 17-ketosteroid hormone content of adrenal gland could not account for the increased urinary output of the hormone:

Kuhn and Knuchel found that 5 to 8 mg of 17-ketosteroids are applied per 100 to 150 mg of lyophilized adrenal gland tissue. However, the increased daily urinary output of 17-ketosteroids over a period of several weeks following the injection ranged between 8 and 9 mg. They were right to conclude that the amount of hormones injected was by no means sufficient to account for the increased output. Therefore we are not dealing with a substitution, but rather with an activation of an intensifying mechanism, about which we know little.

(Schmid and Stein, 1967)

In a current commercially available preparation such as Standard Process Desiccated Adrenal,® the amount of adrenal gland is 130 mg per tablet. This tablet size is in the same range as the amounts used by the above authors.

Schmid continues with this thesis, "In addition, the results of studies by NEUMANN (1954), BERNHARD and KRAMPITZ (1957), STRUM (1955), KUHN and KNUCHEL (1954), KNUCHEL (1955) and other authors are incompatible with the concept that the hormones contained in the transplanted (injected) tissue could explain the effects of cellular therapy" (Schmid and Stein, 1967).

As each hormone was isolated and synthesized, the injectable gland cell product was taken out of general medical use and discussion removed from texts like the American Medical Association publications on drugs and other medical treatments (*American Medical Association,* 1916, 1946). The misconception that substituting for the glands' function was somehow equal to or better than the administration of gland cell preparation aimed at rebuilding the function of the gland is devastating to the recovery of patients who want to remain without dependence on synthetic hormones for life. Because of this error, ordinary medicine uses these suppressive synthetic hormones as its only treatment for glandular weakness.

The real use of these isolated, synthetic substances should be limited to substitution therapy at the time of complete glandular failure. A Type 1 diabetic needs insulin to survive. A woman with surgical menopause at an early age needs to replace ovarian hormones. A person with thyroid cancer, which makes the complete removal of the gland necessary, must have hormone replacement therapy to avoid serious ramifications.

In each of these cases, there is no possibility of stimulating the gland to function normally. In addition, there is no danger of decreasing the function of the gland through suppression, by substituting for its function. In these cases, the administration of hormones is prudent and safe.

Each gland chapter gives references to sources of glandular material and their dose so the practitioner can compare glandular sources to make an informed decision about the amount of a glandular material to administer in any situation.

Unfortunately, injectable glandular preparations are difficult to obtain in the United States, and their legality is somewhat in question. Because of these facts, we must rely on oral administration of gland cell therapy products.

As recently as the 1940s, every major drug manufacturer in the United States produced these injectable materials (Wolf, 1940). Many companies continued for years after. These materials are widely available in Europe and Mexico at very reasonable prices.

Combination Glandular Products

The use of combination products in gland cell therapy has been popular for many years. These combinations contain the animal gland and often herbs or synthetic vitamins known to help build or nourish the gland. If you use these products, keep some facts in mind. The manufacturer chose, usually for reasons not known to the practitioner, certain vitamins or minerals, to add to a gland substance to enhance the effect of the gland material. This is a problem because it prevents the individual practitioner from choosing the right combination of elements to treat the patient holistically. It is better to choose whole foods for the vitamin and mineral content you want to give and select only the individual gland material that each patient needs.

The only time to select a readymade formulation is through personal experience with that formula and research into the reasons for each ingredient's inclusion in the formula. Integrative endocrinology demands selection of individual ingredients for each case, not the use of prepared combination products, which often contain synthetic vitamins or herbal extracts that may not be appropriate for every patient.

Gland cell therapy is the premiere method for treating the endocrine system. The gland causing the patient's trouble can be targeted easily, and the exact nutrients needed in the exact combination and amounts needed by the gland for rebuilding are all present.

5 Manipulative Therapy

The best-known and most-practiced manipulative therapy in current use is chiropractic. There are many styles now; some adhere to the principles of the founder, and some do not. The underlying philosophical framework of chiropractic is to manipulate the bones, particularly of the spine, to free the nerves to allow free flow of nerve energy and blood supply.

Assessing the dysfunction known as subluxation and correcting it returns tone to the system, allowing healing to take place. From an endocrine standpoint, spinal adjustment may aid the case tremendously. Manipulative therapy treats the nerve and blood supply to the various glands. It does not treat the gland directly.

D. D. Palmer, founder of chiropractic, wrote,

> On September 18, 1895, Harvey Lillard called upon me. He was so deaf for seventeen years that he could not hear the noises on the street. Mr. Lillard informed me that he was in a cramped position and felt something give in his back. I replaced the displaced 4th dorsal vertebra by one move, which restored his hearing fully.
>
> (Palmer, 1910)

This was Palmer's initial experience of spinal adjustment.

The origin of the word is interesting. Chiropractic comes from *chir* (o) Gr. *cheir*, hand + Gr. *prassein*, to do (Dorland's, 2003).

As Palmer explained, "The activity of these nerves, or rather their fibers, may become excited or allayed by impingement, the result being a modification of functionating—too much or not enough action—which is disease" (Palmer, 1910).

Palmer believed the cause of all disease is a change in nerve function. With function restored, the disease no longer exists and the body can begin the healing process. This explanation of disease seems simplistic when seen with our current knowledge. However, observing from the viewpoint of clinical experience, this explanation is often accurate.

Using chiropractic adjustment as an aid to healing the endocrine glands is a great adjunct to oral treatments like herbs, nutrition, or gland cell therapy. The adjustment can help the nutritional aspects of these treatments to enter the gland by opening the nerve and blood circulation to the area.

An integrative endocrine team must have a chiropractor. Although adjustments are usually done with the hands, a chiropractor may use a handheld device like the "activator" or props like hip blocks from sacral–occipital technique.

Another important manipulative device is the Manaka wooden hammer (Manaka and Birch, 1995). This is a small wooden hammer with a leather striking surface and a small peg. The peg is set in contact with a point on the body and struck lightly with the hammer.

It is easy to make a Manaka hammer using a small wooden hammer and a dowel. The dowel is 0.5 inch in diameter, with the patient contact end cut down to 0.25 inch and rounded to a smooth end. The dowel is about 3 inches long. The patient can use this device at home. If using this device at acupuncture points, then a specific frequency for each meridian is used. The frequency is set by listening to a metronome and following the rhythm when the acupuncture point corresponds to a meridian as shown in Figure 5.1.

Only 20 beats per point is used, but at the frequency of the meridian (Manaka, 1995).

The other technique from Dr. Manaka is to have the patient listen to the metronome sound for the meridian affected without using the tapping hammer while acupuncture points related to the affected gland are stimulated by hand.

Manaka used a Seiko electronic metronome (Model DM 70) that also generates all 12 musical tones. You may also select the pitch that relates to the gland you are treating to add sound therapy. These metronomes are inexpensive and very easy for the patient to use at home. This technique is an interesting cross of acupuncture, manipulative therapy, and sound therapy.

If you are trying to mobilize a vertebral level by tapping the muscle adjacent to the vertebra or on or between the spinous processes, then the frequency is not so important.

The Manaka technique is very similar to Spondylotherapy, invented by Dr. Albert Abrams (Abrams, 1910). Abrams used a piece of linoleum 6 inches long, 1.5 inches wide, and 0.25 inch thick. Put the linoleum in contact with the skin and strike it lightly with a hammer. Direct the percussion to the spinous process of the vertebra requiring the adjustment. The hammer is similar to a Bucks neurological hammer. Unlike the Manaka technique, no particular rhythm is essential.

Yin Channels	Beats
Ren mai	104
Lung	126
Spleen	132
Heart	126
Kidney	120
Pericardium	176
Liver	108
Yang Channels Du Mai	104
Large Intestine	108
Stomach	132
Small Intestine	120
Bladder	112
Triple Burner	152
Gall Bladder	120

Figure 5.1 Manaka Metronome Chart.

Osteopathy is another manipulative therapy introduced into practice in 1874 by its founder, Andrew Taylor Still (1828–1917). The basic premise of osteopathy is that restoring nerve and blood supply can cure conditions distant from the area of manipulation.

In modern America, the osteopaths are completely absorbed by ordinary medicine so that osteopaths graduating now are fully licensed physicians and surgeons. This means that they may prescribe all drugs and do all other forms of medical practice just as medical doctors can. Very few of the currently graduating osteopaths practice as Dr. Still did. If you are thinking about an osteopathic referral, ask questions to make sure that the practitioner fits your patient's needs.

Any of these forms of manipulative therapy will be of great assistance to the endocrine system. Opening the blood circulation and nerve pathways to the glands, they can function at a higher level. Delivering nutrients and removing toxins with adequate blood supply will allow each gland to function at maximum efficiency. The use of manipulative therapy in an integrative endocrine case will make all other therapies more effective.

6   Nutrition

The problem with nutrition is, no one is telling the truth. The foods that are making Americans fat and sick are the foods of commerce, that is, refined grains, corporate meat, raised with hormones and antibiotics, high fructose corn syrup, dairy products that are not whole or raw, and soy products.

Corporate conglomerates produce the foods of commerce. These are huge farms with multiple locations. The problem of corporate-produced food, not truthfully labelled, has existed since the inception of the Food and Drug Administration (FDA).

The first head of the FDA, Dr. Harvey Wiley, confiscated bleached flour in 1910. The court case lasted until 1919, travelling to the Supreme Court and back to the original court for retrial. The manufacturer lost the case, and the government destroyed the flour. Unfortunately, the case did not change the practice of bleaching the flour.

Removing the wheat germ and bleaching dramatically increases the shelf life and strips almost all nutritional value except carbohydrate content. Manufacturers then add synthetic vitamins, manufactured from coal tar derivatives, to enrich the flour. This is a perfect recipe for tissue degeneration and obesity.

Not surprisingly, Wiley did not last long as the head of the FDA. Wiley documented his experiences in a book, *The History of a Crime against the Food Law,* in 1929.

The same problems Wiley documented were also outlined by Alfred W. McCann in *Starving America,* (1913), *The Science of Eating* (1918), and *The Science of Keeping Young* (1926). The copyright on all these books changed hands and they could not be reprinted after the death of the authors, thereby suppressing the information (Lee, 1950). Although the information in these books is dated, they point out that a battle has been raging since the beginnings of American corporate food production between corporate food producers interested in profit and those interested in long-term health effects of food.

Modern food production increases shelf life and uses food that is easy to produce. This has decreased diversity in the American diet and increased corporate profits. The results of this battle are all to the nutritional detriment of the American public.

Even in the latest publication from The Endocrine Society and The Hormone Foundation titled *The Endocrine Society Weighs In, A Handbook on Obesity in America*, these facts are not discussed and a real solution is not offered. Many statistics are quoted about the rampant obesity in America. The society recognizes the problem and is in a unique position to offer solutions. With 11,000 members, it could have a dramatic voice in shaping policy in America, but no real concrete solutions are in the book.

For practitioners, one of the difficulties with nutrition is organizing your thinking for each individual patient's problem. Dr. Bernard Jensen, one of the author's long-time mentors and teaching associates, solved this problem in one way, and Dr. Royal Lee, founder of the Standard Process Company, solved it in another way.

Jensen solved the problem with information he learned from V.G. Rocine. Jensen always referred to Rocine as a Norwegian homeopath; however, in the volume *Brief Biographical Sketch of V.G. Rocine*, authored by his wife, only mentioned are his Swedish boyhood and many generations of his family in French nobility. His teaching and books center more on nutrition and right living, not homeopathy.

During a time in 1988 when I lived with Jensen at his ranch in Escondido, California, there for the purpose of reading and providing an analysis of 500 iris photos that had been taken at his 80th birthday celebration that September, I had full access to his personal library for several months. During this time, I came across copious notebooks of mimeographed papers from his study with V.G. Rocine. When asked if I could copy these notes, Jensen replied that all the information in the notes he had put into his book, *The Chemistry of Man*.

The basic idea presented in this volume is that every tissue and organ in the body has an affinity for one or several chemical elements that are contained in the food we eat. With a proper diagnosis of the tissues involved in a person's ailment, the practitioner can prescribe a diet that contains the foods high in the needed elements so the body may go about the business of healing.

Two examples: the stomach is a sodium organ, meaning that the stomach tissue contains a lot of sodium compared to other organs. If the stomach is ailing in some way, it is lacking this vital element; so feeding high sodium foods will help in healing. These are foods naturally high in bioavailable sodium, not added salt. Some of these foods: goat milk or cheese, goat whey powder, sunshine fruits like oranges or grapefruit, or vegetables like okra and many others. The skin is a silica tissue. Giving foods high in silica will aid the healing of skin, hair, and nail tissues. Silica foods include the peels of fruits and vegetables (leave them on if possible), flax seeds, oat straw tea, and tincture of Avena sativa.

Jensen used iridology for his diagnostic technique. Iridology is very effective and useful, but not necessary in all cases. For example, skin ailments are usually obvious. A differential diagnosis is unnecessary to begin treatment with silica foods and have a successful outcome.

Lee took another approach. He used the tissue from animals that matched the diseased tissue in the patient. The idea has been in use since the beginning of written medical history. The method, described by Hippocrates, Galen, Paracelsus, and Pliny the Elder, was the basis of endocrinology until 1921 with the isolation of insulin, the first mass-produced hormone.

That discovery started a revolution in endocrinology that promoted substitution of the function of the various hormonal outputs of glands as superior to applying nutrition to heal the gland both functionally and structurally.

Lee went a step further and perfected a way to use just the nucleus of the cell in his supplements instead of the whole cell, thereby introducing the growth factors without all the other elements contained in the cell. This process is the basis for what he called protomorphology. It is nearly identical to the modern process of oral tolerance (Weiner, 2004), except that the new method does not use just the nuclear portion of the cell, and consequently, does not achieve results equal to Dr. Lee.

A review of Lee's 1947 book *Protomorphology* clearly reveals that the protomorphogen is the mineral skeleton of protein. The intravenous injection of a 10 percent saline solution of this material obtained by ashing a protein at 300 °C will produce death if given to the same species of animal as the original tissue. "The hypothetical mineral protomorphogen solution is postulated to serve as a framework upon which organic components are assembled into an antigenetically active foreign protein. The serologic reaction therefore is against this protein and not directly against the ash itself" (Fishbein, 1948). What Lee has given and the reviewer accurately describes, but fails to perceive, is an explanation for autoimmune disease. The ash, when injected forms a protein around itself and the body mounts an immune response. The reviewer continues, "to follow their further discussion and elaboration would not serve a useful purpose" (Fishbein, 1948).

Not only did the reviewer miss the point of the creation of an autoimmune disease, but also the possibility of the treatment of autoimmune conditions with something as simple as the tissues of animals that matched the tissue in a human disease condition.

Lee's fundamental work is really the beginning of oral tolerance, the most promising treatment for autoimmunity today. It is also possibly one explanation for why the administration of glandular products from animals heals the glands of humans.

Nutrition is the foundation of any integrative endocrinology program.

The closer the diet is to organic, the better effect it will have on the glandular system. Organic food is healthier. It did not need the help of pesticides or herbicides or fertilizers to be a healthy plant or animal. The organic method provides a more nutritious and energetically viable product. Eating entirely organic is not always possible in every situation, but the more it can be done, the less work the body must do to eliminate any foreign materials that comes with the food.

Many of the substances we ingest with our food are xeno-hormones. These may come from the plants themselves, like soy acting as a xeno-estrogen, from an actual hormone used in raising livestock to petrochemicals and plastics that can block hormone receptor sites not allowing the real hormone to act on that site. These foreign materials are endocrine disruptors.

Suggestions in each gland chapter are made for certain foods or vitamins, minerals and other nutrients. The suggestions are specific to that gland. These foods should be from as whole, raw, and natural a source as possible. The idea of nutrition in relation to endocrinology is to provide foods that help the rebuilding of specific glands to aid the more specific measures in the overall plan for the individual patient.

The problem of endocrine disruptors is increasingly evident to scientists and is now being widely reported in the news media. Studies of endocrine disruptors show a definite effect on the receptor sites for various hormones caused by intake of plastics. The main source is the use and reuse of plastic bottles for food and beverages. The companies producing these products are attempting to confuse the situation by conducing studies of the same materials to show that they are toxic only at very high concentrations. It takes very small amounts of these materials to alter the function of the endocrine system but very high amounts to kill you. These are very different studies with very different parameters and outcomes.

It is reported that women with small amounts of fermented soy in their diets, like Oriental women, are not affected by menopausal symptoms, whereas women who use isoflavones extracted from soy and taken as nutritional supplements, do not get the same benefit. This is another example of the problem of mistaking one active ingredient as the prime reason why a food or other nutrient such as a herb has a specific effect in humans.

Why has Marinol® not had the clinical success of medical marijuana? Why didn't the Szent-Gyorgyi experiments with crystalline vitamin C yield the same excellent results as his experiments with Hungarian paprika? These are questions of extracted partial nutrients and not the whole food. This author believes that foods and herbs should be as whole, raw, and natural as possible.

A few general dietary guidelines are helpful to anyone and particularly those with endocrine difficulties. One of our main objectives is to keep the blood glucose levels balanced. Eating a balance of protein, fat, and carbohydrate in approximately one-third portions most easily does this.

Diabetic patients need some more specific adjustments, especially to increase protein. All diabetic changes should be based on blood sugar measurements.

Another key to balanced blood glucose levels is paying attention to the glycemic index of foods. A simple chart of the glycemic index of foods should be given to the patient with the instruction to eat with a tendency to the lower glycemic index foods. These foods digest more slowly and have less sugar content.

Whole grains are lower on the scale than refined grains. Vegetables have a varying level with potatoes and carrots being high glycemic index and foods like spinach, lettuce, and broccoli being lower on the scale.

The proteins should be organic if possible. Animal protein in the diet is one way that hormones, not intended for the person, might be inadvertently ingested from commercially produced livestock. Antibiotics and other drugs used in animal husbandry may also be present in nonorganic meat.

The fats should be from a whole food source. Olive oil, butter, avocado, eggs, and coconut oil are best. Some patients may be concerned about dietary cholesterol. Keep in mind that most of the major hormones depend on cholesterol as a precursor and removing dietary cholesterol only lowers the serum cholesterol about 10 percent to 15 percent at most (Guyton and Hall, 2000).

In addition, when decreasing dietary cholesterol, the liver detects the change and, in a feedback loop, will begin to produce more endogenous cholesterol than before the dietary change (Guyton and Hall, 2000). Treating the liver and reducing the simple carbohydrate intake will lower serum cholesterol much more effectively than reducing dietary cholesterol.

Preparing your own food is best. Anytime commercially prepared food is used, you are getting many additives and preservatives that have no food value and may be harmful to you. The harm may be minimal, but these are still byproducts that must be metabolized and eliminated from the body.

For support of any system in the body, especially the glands, do not take synthetic vitamins or nutrients that have been extracted from their whole food material or that are laboratory creations. Using whole foods or whole food supplements that contain a high amount of nutrients will allow the body to extract the nutrients it needs to build healthy tissue for the glands and other tissues.

In addition, all the co-factors needed to properly metabolize these nutrients will be present in whole foods and whole food supplements. This creates a nutritional as opposed to a pharmacological approach to healing the gland. Using synthetic or isolated nutrients, that is, vitamin C as ascorbic acid, in large doses, which typically can be 1 to 5 grams or more per day, creates a pharmacological effect in the body. A secondary depletion of nutrients takes place, in this case the bioflavinoids, which help vitamin C to be used in the body as a nutrient.

Food as whole, raw, and natural is best.

7   Western Herbal Medicine

The model for using Western herbs is ordinary or conventional medicine. This is true because ordinary medicine springs from the practice of herbal medicine as practiced by Hippocrates and Galen with synthetic or semisynthetic drugs used in place of plant- or animal-based medicines. Western, or perhaps more properly European, herbal medicine is practiced in the way that a single medicinal plant or a simple combination is used for a single body area or clinical problem. This style of prescribing is as old as humanity and, in some cases, it even extends into the animal kingdom.

The idea that animals can select herbs for their own healing is common in folklore traditions, even in relatively modern-day America. Harry Hoxsey, creator of the famous Hoxsey herbal cancer treatment, stated many times that his grandfather watched a sick horse with a tumor select certain plants to eat when left in a field to die. The horse lived and the grandfather started collecting the herbs revealed by the horse and administered them to other animals and people, supposedly curing many and giving his grandson the ability to start some of the largest cancer treatment centers in the United States.

The Bible even contains stories of herbs used for the treatment of medical conditions.

In Western civilization, women passed down herbal remedies through many generations and, in 1902, Benedict Lust took these herbal remedies, the use of nutrition, water therapy, sunlight, and exercise, and founded the practice of naturopathy. The philosophy of naturopathy is to use the healing power of nature (*vis medicatrix naturea*) as the main driving force for the treatment of human ailments.

There are many forms used for administering herbal medicines. The most fundamental method is to steep the herb in a cup of hot water to make a tea. This is an infusion. The hot water extracts some of the water-soluble medicinal properties from the herb and delivers them to the body in a form that is easy to assimilate. The other water extraction method is a decoction that involves leaving the herbs in simmering water for a longer time. This allows for the extraction of more of the medicinal power of the herb.

Another way to take herbs with minimal processing is to grind the herb into a powder and place it into a capsule, relying on the digestive process to extract the medicinal properties, instead of just hot water.

The medicinal properties are extracted from herbs by using other substances that break down the cellular structure of the plant and release its healing properties. The usual solvent is ethyl alcohol. This form of medicinal substance, called a tincture, requires some precision in processing. Some of the medicinal effects of herbs are released by water and others by alcohol, so the percent combination of alcohol and water is important in releasing the maximum medicinal effect into the tincture. These exact percentages, used for many years, are available in all reputable herbal books and medical pharmacopeias of the past as listed in the Reading List. Other extracting solvents are glycerin and various oils.

The administration of each herb is dependent on its strength and method of manufacture. The practitioner must take care to understand the manufacturer's potency to know the correct dose. Using an herb as a simple tea may render the dose somewhat imprecise. The dose of a fine powder in a capsule requires more attention from the prescriber. Dose ranges for raw herbs can vary widely. Adjustment of the dose is necessary if the manufacturer uses a concentrating process of the whole herb or the tincture process.

This author prefers to use herbs in tincture form. Removing all the cellulose makes the medicinal properties more readily absorbed into the body, with a minimum of digestion.

This author strongly disagrees with a practice beginning to creep into the herbal marketplace. Let's call it the active ingredient fraud. Someone decides—by legitimate experimentation or otherwise—that a certain ingredient in a herbal preparation is responsible for its medicinal action in the body. Then comes a decision about how much of this ingredient produces the medicinal effect. Support for this dose level supposedly comes from researchers or experiments to add legitimacy. Often, there is no consideration given to dose. A product is created that contains many times the amount of the supposed active ingredient than is in the whole herb. This ingredient no doubt has an effect on the human body, but is it *the* effect?

Standardization is the process of adding the active ingredient of a herb in a higher potency than it occurs naturally. The so-called active ingredient is extracted from a quantity of the herb. Another batch of the same herb is tested for the amount of active ingredient it contains. The previously extracted active ingredient is now added to the new batch to make the herb contain exactly the predetermined amount of active ingredient per patient dose. The reason for this procedure is to give the appearance of pharmaceutical precision to herbal medicine and to dramatically increase the one ingredient.

The problem with this method is the balance of constituents originally in the herb as it grew in nature is now altered. If herbs, used for thousands of years to heal without manipulation, have their essential nature changed in the laboratory, what is the result?

This is how Western pharmacology originated. If you continue to refine a so-called active ingredient and exclude all other plant substances, you get an extremely medicinally active compound. With high medicinal activity comes the specter of the side effect.

A plant draws to itself the chemical elements that make it what it is. By virtue of the plant's genetics, the soil, the water, and the sunshine to produce photosynthesis, a plant has a chemical makeup or biochemical signature. This unique composition of elements gives the plant certain attributes when used as a medicine. In the human body, the elements in the plant work together to create a synergistic effect. Many of the substances contained in herbal medicines creating a physiologic effect in the body are known. Many of the substances are unknown.

Herbs in their whole state bring with them all the necessary factors and cofactors with the whole plant. Few side effects are seen with herbal medicine when used in this manner. In the standardized herbal product, the active ingredient is in an imbalanced proportion to the rest of the ingredients. Nutraceutical is another name for these standardized herb products. The name reveals that they are half nutritional, half pharmaceutical.

Opium is a good example from the plant kingdom with well-known actions and a very long history. The dried exudate of the plant is either smoked or taken orally. The morphine content of opium is no less than 7.5 percent.

Elaborating on the previously mentioned point, standardization of opium could be like deciding that morphine was the active ingredient in opium and standardizing opium to contain 50 percent morphine by adding pure morphine back into raw opium. This would have a much more powerful, unpredictable, and untested effect as compared to the originally produced pure opium.

Standardization is very different from the herbology practiced in the past. The perceived pharmacologically active ingredient is in a higher dose, while the other nutrient material of the herb is reduced in these standardized products. This author believes that standardized herbs are more akin to pharmacology, not the usual nutritive effect of true herbal medicine.

Shamanism offers another view of herbal prescribing (Cowan, 1995). Each plant has an individual nature, its own intrinsic energy, or an innate intelligence. If we change this by extracting, concentrating, and reconstituting, which some kind of research has shown to be beneficial, we are practicing Western pharmacology, not herbal medicine. The native healers in the Western part of the state of Montana in the United States recognize this innate intelligence in plants. When they select a plant remedy for an individual patient they do not do so because a plant is known to be good for a certain condition as in European-based herbology. The shaman forages in the forest with the individual patient in mind and selects the herb that reveals itself to the shaman as helpful for the individual in question. The shaman perceives the individual nature of the plant and compares it to the individual nature of the patient.

This perspective has a lot in common with the practice of homeopathy. The homeopath selects a remedy based on the symptoms produced by the remedy when given to a healthy person, the innate intelligence of the remedy, and the individual symptoms of the patient regardless of the cause of the symptoms.

Each gland chapter will give instructions for the dose of raw herb to use and a dose schedule. In addition, as far as possible, there are instructions for the use of tinctures, herb capsules, or water or glycerin extracts.

8   Neural Therapy

Neural therapy is the injection of procaine (trade name: Novocain) into affected areas of the body. Albert Einhorn first synthesized procaine in 1905 while searching for a local anesthetic without the psychic effects of cocaine. The ingredients of procaine are para amino benzoic acid (PABA) and diethylaminoethanol (DEAE). It is almost completely metabolized without affecting the liver, a unique quality among local anesthetics.

Procaine was used only as a local anesthetic until 1925 when Ferdinand and Walter Huneke discovered its curative effects. The reason procaine has a healing effect on many conditions, including imbalances in the glandular system, is its effect on the potassium/sodium pump at the cellular level. A cell becomes depolarized for many reasons. Depolarization takes place when a constant stimulus, such as toxins or an unhealed injury, causes potassium to leave the cell and sodium to enter the cell and remain in this state. Depolarization is a change in the membrane potential of the cell that makes the cell membrane permeable and thus open to further injury and decreased function.

Applying a local anesthetic seals the cell by turning off the potassium/sodium pump, causing an increased internal cellular metabolism. The cell, because of the increased metabolism, is able to expel the sodium and take in more potassium, reestablishing its membrane potential and ridding itself of toxins. This action brings the cell back to a healthy state.

There are three applications of neural therapy for hormonal imbalances. The first method is the injection of 1 cc of procaine 2% intravenously. This injection has a harmonizing effect on the entire glandular system. The second application is injecting procaine directly into the glands, such as the thyroid, adrenal, or prostate. Third, you may inject into a related point when the gland is not accessible such as acupoint GV (Governing Vessel) 20 for the pituitary gland.

For each gland, you may select the neural therapy point or the related acupuncture point for injection, or both. Injecting procaine into the appropriate acupuncture point for each individual gland can be a very effective approach. Using this method, you do not need to be as accurate as when using an acupuncture needle.

That procaine is a prescription medicine limits its use to qualified practitioners. National organizations that train neural therapists maintain referral lists, so adding this modality to a team approach is possible.

Many injection sites used for neural therapy are the same as acupuncture points. In addition, many points of pain described by patients are also acupuncture points. A thorough study of the indications of the acupuncture points for each indicated glandular condition will be helpful in giving an effective neural therapy treatment.

Mathias Dosch MD, author of the two main texts of neural therapy, shares this author's view of hormone replacement therapy:

> If we give our patient hormonal preparations to replace his/her own, the feedback system signals that the hormonal levels are adequate or even excessive, and the body's own production is consequently further reduced instead of being stimulated. If treatment continues long enough, the organism will altogether cease producing these hormones. The regulatory dysfunction is then moved to other control circuits, and thus makes it possible for secondary disorders to arise there. Hence, the systems become iatrogenically unstable and more labile instead of healthier. Our task is to unblock them and make them again capable of reacting, in order to enable the spontaneous healing powers to function again as far as possible and to remain permanently functional.
>
> (Dosch, 1984)

Dr. Ana Aslan, of Romania, also found very interesting properties of procaine. She claimed that using intravenous injections, intramuscular injections, and oral administration of pills had an effect on aging. She also found, during many years of research in gerontology, a very positive effect on chronic problems such as arthritis. Her procaine compound called Gerovital H3 continues to be available. GH-3 is slightly different from ordinary procaine in that it is more acidic with a pH of 3.3. It is possible that the antiaging effects Aslan found were the same gland-regulating effects reported by the neural therapists.

Neural therapy, according to Huneke, as this practice is formally known, is a much more complex system than presented here. The information in this chapter is adapted for integrative endocrinology only and omits the much more expansive ways in which neural therapy is used in a myriad of other conditions.

9   Color Therapy

Color therapy is the application of specific frequencies of the visible portions of the electromagnetic spectrum to the body. There are many methods to apply color therapy. Use of a lamp made for this purpose is one of the most popular and effective. Shining a colored light on a container of water and then drinking the water is another popular method. Wearing clothing of a particular color creates that color's frequency vibration on a selected area of the body. Using meditative techniques accomplishes the same purpose.

Color therapy uses the visible light frequencies of the electromagnetic spectrum. These visible frequencies do not have the same destructive characteristics as the frequencies that are just outside the visible spectrum. The frequencies just outside the visible spectrum are ultraviolet, with its skin-burning potential and bactericidal properties, or infrared, with its heat-producing qualities.

There are two separate and distinct forms of color therapy in general use today. One of these forms comes from the East Indian yoga traditions that assign a color to each chakra. Each chakra connects to a specific endocrine gland and then to a spinal level. A chakra is an energy center existing outside the physical body. The seven chakras are rooted to the physical body by the seven main endocrine glands. This form of color application is somewhat vague in its selection of color frequencies. For example, detecting a thyroid disorder or a throat chakra disorder, the color blue is applied to the throat area, but the exact frequency of blue is not generally specified.

One of the main proponents of this type of therapy in modern times was Edwin S. Babbitt (1828–1905). He produced color jars that he called the chromo lens. These had the appearance of a small round flask holding approximately eight fluid ounces. The jars, sold in a variety of colors, each had its own healing properties. The patient hangs the water-filled jar outside on a line in the sunlight. The sunlight instilled the healing properties of the color into the water. Drinking the water gives the healing effect.

Babbitt's book is commonly available today but is unfortunately incomplete, as the editor, in 1967, decided some parts were outdated. This author believes it is the reader's responsibility to make that determination in regards to a classic work.

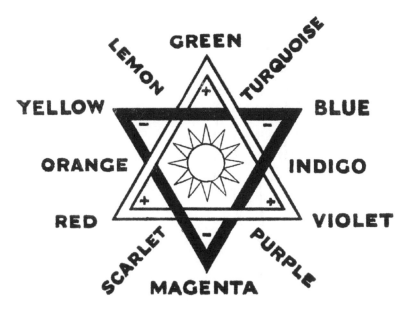

Figure 9.1 Twelve Color Spectro-Chrome System.

Many other authors have written about this particular form of color therapy. Many books exist on using this method with a variety of explanations and techniques. In each gland chapter, you will find the general color for each gland from this method, herein called the chakra method.

A contrasting view of color therapy is from Dinshah P. Ghadiali (1873–1966), always referred to as Dinshah. His system, called spectrochrometry, used what he called attuned color waves. His method of defining these exacting color frequencies was to look at the spectrum and find the numerical center of each color. In this way, the 12 colors he used had a known and exact frequency.

Dinshah separated the body into a number of distinct areas (Figure 9.2) for tonations, as he called the administration of colored light to the surface of the body. Each color and body area is described in each gland chapter.

Dinshah also relied on the variant breath chart to decide the best time of day to tonate a certain body region. This chart is available from the Dinshah Health Society yearly if you are a member. You can calculate your own chart. If you are using this color method on a difficult condition and it is not working well, using the tonation time as calculated by the variant breath chart may be just the right boost.

To calculate variant breath times, start at sunrise and count forward 2 hours and 56 minutes. This is the time of the first 1-hour tonation of that day. Calculate the start times for the whole day by counting these intervals from sunrise every day. Each interval is 2 hours and 56 minutes from the

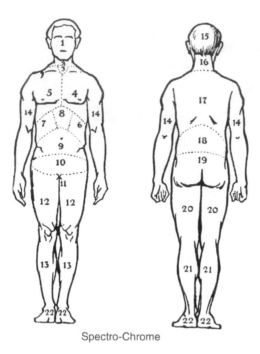

Spectro-Chrome

Figure 9.2 Area Charts.

previous start time. The basis of the breath chart is ancient yogic writing and meditation/breathing tradition.

The original Dinshah color projector had a very powerful 2000-watt lamp. The 12 spectrochrome colors were produced by shining the 2000-watt lamp through a combination of five colored glass slides placed in front of the light. The patent for Dinshah's lamp is available on the Internet: U.S. patent number 1,544,973, July 7, 1925. This patent is a very interesting piece of medical history. Branded as fraudulent many years ago, the machines and all Dinshah's books were ordered destroyed. In fact, in 1950s New Jersey, the machines were destroyed and the books burned. That such a thing could happen in the United States to a man and his obviously effective therapy is horrendous.

The Dinshah Heath Society is still providing Dinshah's original color therapy books and materials, including a variant breath forecast for all areas of the world. They also have a set of plans for building an inexpensive color projector using Roscolene filters (Dinshah, 1985). These filters are for lighting in theaters and can create the exact attuned color waves if used in the right combination. This makes color therapy easy for the practitioner or the patient to use with minimal expense. The numbers of the Roscolene® filters that need to be used together to create the spectrochrome colors are shown in Table 9.1.

Table 9.1 Roscolene® Filter Numbers for Spectrochrome Slides.

Spectrochrome color	Roscolene® filters
Red	818+828
Yellow	809
Green	871
Blue	859+866
Violet	832+859+866
Magenta	818+828+866
Orange	809+828
Lemon	809+871
Turquoise	861+871
Indigo	828+859+866
Purple	832+866
Scarlet	810+818+861

The exact instructions from Dinshah's writings appear in each gland chapter, including the color to use and the body area to tonate.

Therapy using visible light may seem, at first glance, a little esoteric. If we can look at another use of light and vibrational frequencies in medicine, it may become less strange. In the science of spectroscopy, a compound is burned and the light given off by the flame is viewed through a spectroscope. A spectroscope is a device that focuses visible light through a prism. As the light is fractioned into its representative unique color pattern, it reveals the chemical elements in the burning material.

Each chemical element has a distinct color signature when viewed in this way. This is the method used to determine the chemical composition of stars. This is also one of the ways of performing a hair mineral and metals analysis. The hair is flamed, the light is directed through a prism, and the spectrum is analyzed to see what elements are giving off their unique signature of color.

Meditation practice is another method of delivering color therapy. The first technique is to visualize the color associated with the endocrine gland at the location of that gland. A concentrated focus is necessary, but for an experienced meditator this is a simple matter.

The second meditation method is a breathing meditation. If the natural world is viewed as the colors of the rainbow, indigo is at the highest heavens, violet is a little lower, blue is the visible sky level, green is at the level of the grass and trees, yellow is at the level of earth, orange is a bit lower and red is at the level of the magma of the volcanic areas of the earth. The color needed is taken in as a breath from the earth area of the respective color. Focus the color inspired with the breath on the appropriate gland. Exhale clear air; leave the color in the gland. In this way, the color of the appropriate gland is concentrated by meditation at the location of the gland. This method effectively brings the color to the glandular area and initiates healing with this powerful method.

10 Chinese Medicinals

This therapy is often misnamed Chinese Herbal Medicine, but the name is not sufficient to describe the actual practice. Chinese internal medicine uses many other substances in addition to herbs, that is, medicinal plants. Common examples of other products are oyster shells, the bones of animals, tissues from animals (e.g., glands), and humans (e.g., placenta), insects (e.g., cicada), and minerals (e.g., cinnabar).

Before prescribing Chinese medicinal products, it is essential to make an appropriate Chinese eight-principle diagnosis. Diagnosis in the Chinese tradition bears little relation to diagnosis in the Western tradition. The main tools are the patient's report of symptoms and the Two Pillars of Oriental diagnosis, observation of the tongue and pulse.

The clinician observes the tongue for changes in its physical structure, and the color of the body of the tongue and the structure and color of its coat. Divisions on the body of the tongue represent the different meridians, and therefore, the different physical and energetic areas of the body.

The appearance of scallops or the impression made by the teeth on the side of the tongue is an indication of weakness or vacuity in the kidney meridian and perhaps the physical kidney itself, which may mean adrenal insufficiency. In Chinese medicine, the adrenal gland is associated with the kidney meridian.

Redness at the tip of the tongue indicates excess or overactivity—also called repletion—in the heart meridian and perhaps in the physical organ of the heart.

The coating of the tongue is also of great importance. If there is a "furry" and yellow discoloration in the mid portion, then the stomach or spleen meridian is not functioning well.

The second pillar is pulse diagnosis. This is a difficult skill to learn and takes years of practice to use as a basis for a treatment plan. The 12 pulses at the radial artery at the wrist directly correspond to the 12 organ meridians of Oriental medicine.

Table 10.1 Pulse Position and Depths for Oriental Pulse Diagnosis

Right Wrist		Left Wrist	
Superficial	*Deep*	*Superficial*	*Deep*
Large Intestine	Lung	Small Intestine	Heart
Stomach	Spleen	Gall Bladder	Liver
Triple Warmer	Pericardium	Bladder	Kidney

Oriental pulse diagnosis uses three positions and two depths on each wrist as shown in Table 10.1 above. The left and right wrists reflect the pulse of different meridians. The character of the pulse, as palpated by the examiner's finger, is a direct reflection of the character of the energy flowing in the meridian represented by that pulse. The examiner's first three fingers touch the wrist of the patient over the radial artery. The first finger makes contact near the styloid process of the radius bone. The other two fingers contact the radial artery in a natural position proximal to the index finger.

The superficial pulse is the first perception of the pulse as pressure is applied to the skin. The method for feeling the deep pulse is to occlude the artery with the examining finger and then slowly raise the finger until the pulse is again perceptible.

There are two basic ways to establish a pulse diagnosis based on the two major schools of thought in Oriental medicine. A description of the five element or Worsley style is in the acupuncture chapter (Chapter 2). The other style, traditional Chinese medicine (TCM), is the method begun in the early days of the Communist revolution in China in the late 1940s and early 1950s. This is the style taught in most American acupuncture schools today.

The five-element tradition allows for a more specific and direct feel for the energy movement in the meridians. The TCM version requires the definition of the pulse as feeling like one of 28 descriptions of the pulse picture to arrive at the appropriate differentiation of syndromes. Some examples of descriptions of these sensations of the pulse are thready, full, empty, like a string of pearls, and other images or metaphors. The appropriate Chinese medicinal formula is prescribed only after Oriental diagnosis is established by the patient's report of symptoms and the observation of the pulse and the tongue.

One of the main differences between prescribing Chinese medicinals and Western herbs is that the Oriental prescription is most often polypharmaceutical. Over millennia, the Oriental pharmacopoeia has evolved to include many substances into a single medicinal formula for a given diagnostic entity. These combinations are often extensive and complex. The formula may be more exactly adjusted on the basis of observation of the symptoms related to pulse and tongue, and also on the basis of the relative experience of the practitioner to make an accurate diagnosis. The practitioner makes a raw medicinal formula at the time of the visit from individual medicinals in percentages determined by the practitioner's diagnosis.

Patent formulas are proprietary blends produced by many different manufacturers in China and many other countries, including the United States. Old standard formulas from the Chinese, Japanese, or Korean pharmacopoeia are the basis of these proprietary blends. Patent medicines are effective for the most commonly found energetic imbalances diagnosed by Oriental medical practitioners.

There have been questions about the purity of some patent formulas coming from China. Some patents have pharmaceutical products in them such as acetaminophen. Some have contaminants like heavy metals. The practitioner can deal with this in two ways. First, the Fratkin book on patents contains tests done on many formulas and lists the contaminants. Second, many patents are now being made in the United States under good manufacturing practices and are fully tested.

The suggestions for Chinese medicinals in this book will not assume a through knowledge of Oriental diagnosis, but will be given from a Western perspective with a few Oriental diagnostic hints to narrow the prescription of a patent formula.

However, an expert in Oriental diagnosis and therapeutics can be invaluable as a referral while treating a difficult endocrine case to prescribe and follow up as a member of the integrative endocrinology team.

11 Sound

Use music in an integrative endocrine program to promote relaxation and relieve stress. The nervous system interprets certain kinds of music as relaxing. Using music for stress relief can be a very individual thing. Not all people respond to certain styles of music in the same way. Suggest this approach to the patient without imposing your personal taste.

An Internet search shows the enormous amount of research done on the effects of music on the endocrine glands and the production of certain hormones. This is also the subject of many books.

Sound is used as a very specific tool in integrative endocrinology. According to Indian yogic and meditative practices, a specific spinal level enervates each endocrine gland and each of these levels corresponds to a chakra, an energy center.

A simple way to stimulate an endocrine gland using sound is to tone the appropriate note with the voice. The gland chapters contain the information on the notes for each chakra and gland. Do this practice in a meditative fashion. The instructions are as follows: Sit in a comfortable position. Breathe in deeply from the abdomen. As you release your breath, tone the note. Then you can focus the note on the area of the body where the gland you are trying to activate is located. Initially, this may be difficult to do for an extended period. With practice a 10- to 15-minute session will be easy. Use any instrument to find the right pitch.

Another way to treat an endocrine gland with sound is using a tuning fork. Set the fork vibrating and then put it in contact with the spinous process of the vertebra that corresponds to the intended gland or hold the fork in contact with the skin over the gland. To amplify this effect, interpose a crystal between the vibrating tuning fork and the body.

To find the appropriate pitch for each note, the Seiko metronome with tone generator is an easier method than tuning forks for the patient to use at home because of the expense involved in procuring the right forks and their availability (see manipulative therapy chapter).

Sound healing is done like a meditative practice for 10 to 15 minutes once or twice a day depending on the severity of the disorder and patient dedication. You will find that an experienced meditator will have fun with this treatment style and be very compliant.

12 Microsystems

A microsystem is any part of the human body, smaller than the whole, that in some way reflects the condition of the entire organism. The smallest of these microsystems is the DNA in the nucleus of the cell. The blueprint of information about the entire organism is contained within the genetic material. In integrative endocrinology, our only access to using this microsystem is by the use of gland cell therapy where we are providing the genetic blueprint to the individual gland cell in an effort to reeducate the cells to form a healthy gland. We can treat the other microsystems directly.

Reflexology

Reflexology is the microsystem of the foot. The fundamental principle is that all areas of the body connect by reflex to the foot. If there is a problem in the adrenal gland, then the area of the foot that corresponds to the adrenal gland will be sore to the touch. This area may also have a deposit that the examiner can feel.

Therapy is by manual pressure on the feet. A treatment from a professional reflexologist takes about 1 hour. Pressure is applied to all areas of the foot in an organized and predetermined format. This system is very popular and finding a practitioner to refer to should be easy. Many of your clients may already be seeing a foot reflexologist. If you share your diagnostic concerns with your patients, they can tell their practitioner to pay special attention to the affected areas. If your patients use reflexology as a self-treatment, you may want to provide a chart and mark the areas you feel warrant special attention. If the patient will work on these areas of the feet for a few minutes every day, they will feel the results.

Two Hand Microsystems

The first hand microsystem is hand reflexology. This is very similar to foot reflexology, but correlation of the positions of the reflex areas is not universal

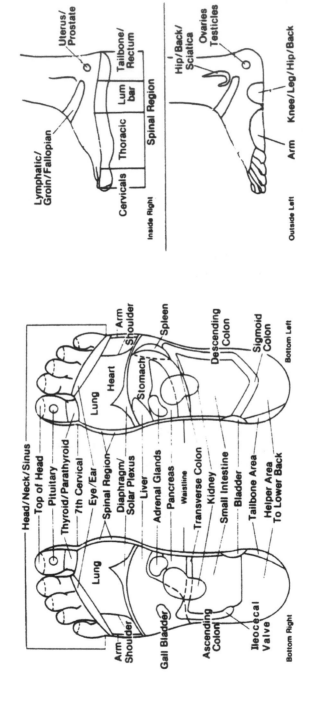

Figure 12.1 Reflexology Chart (by Kevin and Barbara Kunz).

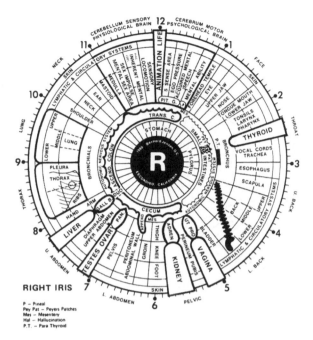

Figure 12.2 Iridology Chart (Right Iris).

as with the foot. No chart is, therefore, included in this text. The second way to use the hand as a reflex or microsystem is the Korean hand acupuncture system of Dr. Tae-Woo Yoo. This system is used with acupuncture needles, pressure, or the beads discussed in the chapter on acupuncture. This is definitely a patient participation modality and a useful adjunct to therapies performed in the clinic. Several charts are available. As with hand reflexology, not all the charts agree.

Iridology

Iridology is included in this chapter because it is one of the premier microsystems. Iridology is the science of observing the iris of the eye to determine changes in the fiber structure (trabeculae) and color to determine the condition of body tissues. The iris of the eye has a reflex to 90 areas of the body just as the whole body is represented by reflex in the microsystem of ear acupuncture (outlined in the acupuncture chapter) and foot or hand reflexology.

The author's work and expertise in iridology comes from 10 years of experience as a teaching associate of Dr. Bernard Jensen and nearly 30 years of clinical experience. Dr. Jensen was the leading authority in the world in the

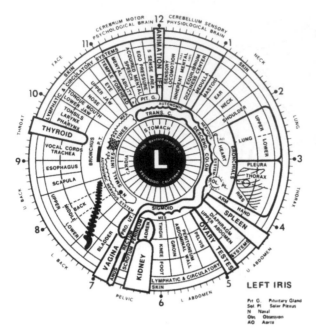

Figure 12.3 Iridology Chart (Left Iris).

practice of iridology and its relation to nutrition. We taught our last class together in June 1992.

The iris analysis is done with magnification by a handheld lens (4x magnification) and light or a specialized camera. The older cameras used photographic slide film, but the newer ones are digital and connect directly to a computer. Many types of practitioners, from herbalists to medical doctors, have used iridology since its inception in 1886. Iridology texts exist in many languages. The originator of iridology was a Hungarian medical doctor. The Germans have done much to advance the practice, particularly with the excellent texts by Josef Deck.

Analysis of all tissues of the body is accomplished through iridology. These are gross structures like the arm or leg or spine and more subtle structures and functions such as the pituitary gland or the animation life center or the five-senses center. According to the tenets of iridology, a direct reflex exists between each of these areas of the body and a very specific area in the iris of the eye.

Observing a specific area in the iris, a direct correlation to the condition of the related tissue is made. There are four basic conditions observed: acute, subacute, chronic, or degenerative.

In the acute phase, the iris fibers are raised and white in color. This means that the organ represented by these fibers is in an inflamed condition. The organ is using nutrients at a high rate and is creating toxins or metabolic waste at a high rate.

In the subacute lesion, the tissue is beginning to be less inflamed and the iris fibers are turning a gray shade instead of white. The normal condition appears somewhere between acute and subacute.

In the chronic state, the iris tissue shows a very definite dark gray tone in a large percentage of the area representing the corresponding tissue.

When a sign in the iris is degenerative, the iris area appears black. No fibers are seen in this area. A degenerative sign indicates the corresponding organ is broken down; it is not letting out toxins or utilizing nutrients.

Iridology is a quick and easy way to make an initial assessment of a glandular case. Iridology will reveal the inherent weaknesses in a person. The practitioner can assess an inherited weakness that is not yet causing any problem. This can allow the practitioner to initiate food choices based on inherited weaknesses in the glandular system so they never become manifest problems. For example, the iris shows a thyroid weakness, but the laboratory tests indicate all values in normal range. Perhaps the person is a bit overweight or cold but no other obvious thyroid symptoms are present. The practitioner can recommend some dietary changes that are helpful to the thyroid. A simple dietary change to benefit the thyroid gland is the use of sea salt or kelp for its dietary iodine content. This can help to build a healthy thyroid function without being specifically therapeutic.

Another wonderful use of iridology in an endocrine case is to assess the relative importance of one compromised gland in relation to others. Is the thyroid subacute and the adrenal chronic or the other way around? This relative analysis can be helpful in directing the importance placed on various treatments or supplements prescribed for that particular patient.

A third distinct advantage in using iridology is it can help the practitioner determine whether a healing program is having a beneficial effect. As each lesion in the iris begins to heal, small white lines begin to form. The greater the healing, the greater the number of these calcium luteum lines. They appear like knitting lines going at angles to the regular lines of the iris fibers.

Iridology is not diagnosis. For example, it can show a chronic or degenerative iris reflex in the pancreas area. This does not tell the practitioner whether the patient has diabetes or an inability to properly form pancreatic enzymes for digestion. The iris sign simply points to a weakness in the pancreas. For a diagnosis of the exact problem, use other methods.

This same lack of Western diagnostic precision is true of the other microsystems. However, they offer a quick and easy way to assess a body imbalance without an invasive procedure and are thus important tools in a holistic approach to endocrinology.

Introduction to Gland Chapters

In this section, we will look at glands generally accepted as part of the endocrine system. We will also be describing organs and structures not normally considered endocrine glands. The reason for this is twofold. First, target tissues that can profoundly affect the glands control many of the mechanisms of the endocrine system. Second, nearly every endocrine text, new and old, contains references to interactions between the endocrines and other organs and tissues. We will, therefore, address some of these issues.

Each gland chapter gives general information about that gland with all chapters having similar subheadings. These chapters are not exhaustive for each gland but rather an introduction to the structure and function that the interested practitioner may use as an initial foray into new areas of research.

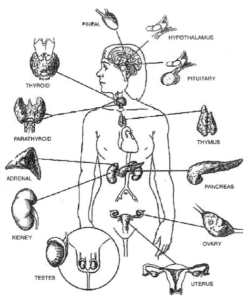

Original Drawing by Diane Ablecff 2002

Location of Endocrine Glands.

Each chapter will outline the specific use of the therapies that are helpful in accomplishing the goal of integrative endocrinology, which is to return the gland and its associated tissues to a state of well-being. If a therapy is not recognized as useful for a certain gland, its subheading is omitted. By understanding the function and interaction of the endocrine glands and related tissues and by using a combination of therapies, you will quickly become successful at the practice of integrative endocrinology.

Reading this section in the order presented, you will notice that the chapters become sparser as you proceed. This occurs because it is not necessary to repeat the information presented in a previous chapter even though it is relevant in every chapter. The lessons learned in any chapter apply equally to all chapters.

All the endocrine glands use a negative feedback loop among the hypothalamus, pituitary, and the target gland whether it is the thyroid, adrenal, ovary, or testicles. The following illustration demonstrates the basic mechanism of this feedback.

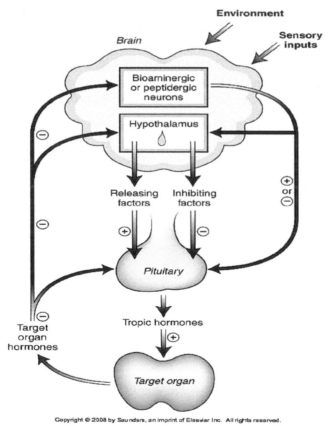

Copyright © 2008 by Saunders, an imprint of Elsevier Inc. All rights reserved.

Regulatory Feedback Loops in Endocrinology.

13 Adrenal Gland

Function and Biochemistry

Location: Above the kidney (suprarenal).

The old books use the picturesque notion of a "cocked hat" on top of the kidney to describe the appearance and location of the gland. The term *suprarenal*, meaning above the kidney, was originally used for humans. In contrast, the term *adrenal*, meaning before or in front of the kidney, is used for animals, because experimentation was first done on animals, whose walking position placed the gland in front of, not on top of, the kidney.

Size: 2 cm wide, 5 cm long, 1 cm thick.

Weight: 4 gm each.

Structure: Comprised of a cortex and medulla. In the adult, the cortex is about 90% of the entire gland. Beneath the external capsule are the following:

- Zona Glomerulosa (ZG)—15% of the cortex
- Zona Fasiculata (ZF)—75% of the cortex
- Zona Reticularis (ZR)—10% of the cortex.

ZF and ZR are completely dependent on ACTH for their structure and function, whereas ZG can function without the pituitary.

The remaining central portion of the adrenal gland is the medulla.

Hormones Produced by the Cortex

- Glucocorticoids (cortisol, cortilsterone)
- Mineralocorticoids (aldosterone, deoxycorticosterone DOC) ZG
- Sex steroids (adrenal androgens, DHEA)

Cholesterol is the precursor of all adrenal steroids. Most is low-density lipoprotein (LDL). This cholesterol is derived from the diet or endogenous synthesis.

Hormones Produced by the Medulla

- Epinepherine (adrenaline)
- Norepinepherine

Functions of Hormones

The glucocorticoids are responsible for modulating metabolism and immune functions.

The mineralocorticoids are responsible for regulation of blood pressure, vascular volume, and electrolytes. Aldosterone is responsible for regulating metabolism of sodium and potassium. The androgens are responsible for appearance of secondary sex characteristics.

Interaction with Other Glands

There is a direct feedback mechanism with the hypothalamus and pituitary. This relationship creates the HPA axis. This interaction has a profound effect on glandular function, so treating only one gland at a time in the HPA axis is often ineffective.

Signs and Symptoms of Disorder or Dysfunction

The medically recognized condition of the insufficiency of the adrenal gland is Addison's disease. This is a disease ultimate or end stage, where the gland has been significantly impacted by a disease process and recovery by natural methods is doubtful. It is said that Addison's is an unusual or rarely seen condition. The condition was originally described by Thomas Addison in a monograph in 1855 titled *On the Constitutional and Local Effects of Disease of the Suprarenal Capsules*. In it he listed the common symptoms of Addison's disease as anemia, general languor and debility, feeble heart action, irritable stomach, with dingy or smokey discoloration of the whole surface of the body, sometimes reaching a deep amber or chestnut brown. Barker later calls these the typical triad of asthenia, disturbance of digestion, and melanoderma (Barker, 1922).

Another view of the same deficiency was offered by Harrower as early as 1917 and is receiving interest in research today. "The most common of the glandular disorders seen in daily practice is fatigue of a chronic nature which is usually due to adrenal insufficiency" (Harrower, 1917). In this instance, Harrower was not meaning the end stage or Addison's, but was referring to a lesser form of the illness causing symptoms, but not leading to death.

Chronic fatigue syndrome (CFS) is often seen as new or a result of our modern age. Harrower in 1922 saw CSF as follows:

Asthenia: The commonest symptom in medicine; Practically all individuals with overburdened systems, that is to say, the majority of cases of chronic disease which are so very common, suffer from aesthenia-loss of strength. In fact, asthenia is probably the commonest single symptom seen in medical practice. The so called "Fatigue Syndrome"—in which the patient tires too easily and too early, in which not only is there muscular tiredness, but initiative is lost and mental capacity is dulled— is one of the most important manifestations in chronic toxemias.

(Harrower, 1922)

This fatigue syndrome is a subclinical hypofunction of the adrenal gland, not as fully developed as Addison's disease. If this syndrome is recognized early, the proper course of integrative endocrinology may be implemented and the gland may be returned to a healthy functioning state. Without treatment, the gland will continue to underfunction and, as is common with the onset of Addison's, during some stress which the weakened adrenal is incapable of handling, succumb to breakdown and an adrenal crisis.

The disease of overactivity of the adrenal glands is Cushing's syndrome. This syndrome is commonly seen when a tumor affects the gland or from the overuse of synthetic adrenal hormonal substances such as prednisone or dexamethazone. The clinical picture of Cushing's syndrome can be dramatic and remarkable in a severe case.

The typical signs are "moon face," truncal obesity, and fat pads in the supraclavicular area and the dorsal cervical area, commonly called a "buffalo hump." Also, striations appear on the abdomen, usually of a purple color. Other symptoms include slender extremities; increased susceptibility to infections, hypertension, renal calculi, osteoporosis, glucose intolerance; and some virilization in females. The stage of Cushing's where many of the above symptoms are present and severe in nature is a disease ultimate and a surgical emergency.

Testing Function

The patient history is extremely important to assess adrenal insufficiency. One of the main symptoms reported is "never well since." For example, after a major surgery, infection, flu, or very stressful life circumstance, the patient complains of not being able to get over colds, flus, or infections. The patient also is unable to recover from stress and has heart palpitations from mild stress situations. The patient may be constantly tired and fatigued from slight exertion. Also they may exhibit chronic morning fatigue.

Here are four simple in-office tests for adrenal insufficiency. The first test is from Dr. Emile Sergent. This was the first article in the very first journal *Endocrinology* published in 1917, produced by The Society for the Study of

Internal Secretions, now known as The Endocrine Society. Dr. Harrower started the society and was editor of the journal so you can see the importance he placed on adrenal fatigue by the article's prominent appearance.

The procedure is to draw a geometric figure on the abdomen of the patient with the finger tip or the dull end of a pen. Care must be taken not to scratch or rub. If a line appears immediately, the pressure has been excessive. After about 30 seconds, a faint line should appear if the reaction is positive for adrenal insufficiency. Eventually the line should exceed the size of the instrument used to produce it. The line should be at its maximum at about 1 minute and remain visible for several minutes.

The second test is known as Ragland's test. This test is a comparison between systolic blood pressure measurements lying down and then quickly standing. In adrenal insufficiency, the blood pressure standing is less than the blood pressure lying. Usually, in a healthy person the systolic pressure will be 4 to 10 mmHg higher standing than sitting.

The third test is for pupillary reactivity. In a darkened room, the patient's pupil is subjected to the light from a penlight shown from the side for 10 seconds. The normal response is for the pupil to remain contracted for the full 10 seconds. If the pupil does not hold its constriction or if the pupil constricts and dilates in a pulsating manner, adrenal hypofunction is assumed (Med. Jour. and Rec., 1924).

The fourth test is to simply observe the pupil of a patient in normal light. This may give some indication of adrenal exhaustion if it is unnaturally dilated. The careful practitioner will compare his observation with the medical history to rule out pharmaceutically induced reaction or the potential of eye injury or disease.

Several laboratory tests may be useful. The easiest test is the 24-hour saliva-free cortisol and dehydroepiandrosterone (DHEA) measurements. There is controversy about the reliability of this test. Some authors state that this test is a more accurate indicator of bioactive hormone levels than blood analysis. Other authors say the opposite. A measurement of unbound levels of cortisol and DHEA is easily obtained in serially collected saliva samples. This gives a picture of the circadian rhythm of the patient in regards to his or her hormone production; conversely, a blood sample shows only the moment the sample is taken. The patient being tested must be functioning at the normal circadian rhythm to make sense of a single-draw blood test. To overcome this problem use serially collected blood samples, if possible. A careful practitioner will continue to follow the literature as new research into the use of these tests is published.

The 24-hour urine hormone profiles are provided by several reference labs. Many hormones and their metabolites are checked by this method. This method is the most accurate and reliable test available. It shows not only the hormones produced by the adrenal and other glands but also the metabolites of the various hormones. The difficulty with the 24-hour urine test is, only the total hormone for 24 hours is known without any knowledge of the circadian rhythm. The rhythm is important because in some patients the rhythm is reversed. To understand this reversal can change treatment decisions in regards to timing of supplementation and strict adherence to a sleep schedule.

See the appendix on pages 143–144 for the hormones and metabolites included in the twenty-four hour urine hormone profile.

Therapy

Acupuncture

In traditional acupuncture theory, the adrenal gland is governed by the kidney meridian.

- K-7 (*Fu Liu*, Returning Current) to tonify the adrenal.
- K-1 (*Yong Quan*, Gushing Spring) to sedate the gland.
- K-10 (*Yin Gu*, Yin Valley) as a supportive treatment is indicated.
- Bl-23 (*Shen Shu*, Back Shu) is the Back-Shu point for the kidney. This point gives direct access to the internal organ and a tonifying or sedating needle manipulation can be given as necessary.
- Gv-4 (*Ming Men*, Gate of Life) this point is below the spinous process of the second lumbar vertebrae and is directly between the Bl-23 points.
- The Voll (Voll, 1978) measurement and treatment point on the trunk is Bl-22.

Obviously, some discrepancies exist between the Voll and Chinese systems, as the Chinese equivalent would be Bl-23 as mentioned above. Where two systems suggest a different approach, palpate both points for pain on pressure, hot or cold sensation, or discoloration to select a point for treatment of the individual patient. The Voll measurement point for the adrenal gland on the extremities is TW-1 (*Guan Chong*, Rushing Past), which can also be used for the gonads.

Auricular Acupuncture

There is surprising agreement between the Chinese system and the French system of Nogier for auricular therapy of the adrenal gland. The adrenal point is "at the lower ridge of the tragus at the very point where it meets the notch" (Nogier, 1972).

Western Herbal Medicine

Licorice (*Glycyrrhiza glabra*). Closely monitor blood pressure when using this herb. "Green Medicine Research Laboratories in Long Island has found active materials in licorice root with a molecular structure similar to that of hormones from the adrenal cortex" (Hutchens, 1973). Dose: 2–6 ml/day of 1:1 liquid extract, 5–15 gm/day of raw herb root, either in bulk as a tea or encapsulated or tablet.

Lobelia *(Lobelia inflata).* "The whole plant is used for critical conditions. The all important adrenal glands are aroused by stimulating adrenalin into the blood stream, it is not accumulative and can be used repeatedly" (Hutchens, 1973). Dose: Low doses stimulate and high doses relax. Use 1 ounce of raw herb in 1 pint of boiled water to make an infusion. The dose is 1 tablespoon, 3 times a day. Lobelia is also available as a tincture or capsule. Follow manufacturers' instructions on dose.

Parsley *(Petroselinum crispum, Apium petroselinum)* is " a specific for the adrenal glands" (Christopher, 1976). 1 ounce raw herb in 1 pint boiled water to make an infusion. The dose is 1 tablespoon, 3 times a day. This will also act as a mild diuretic.

The seven herbs that follow are adaptogenic herbs, that is, they are "helping to conserve adaptation energy as defined in Selye's general adaptation syndrome" (Bone and Mills, 2000). In addition, there is a product recently introduced by Dr. Stephen D. Rogers called Shentrition. This is a powdered mix used to make a shake and is specifically formulated to help with stress and adaptation syndrome.

Chinese Ginseng *(Panax ginseng).* This ginseng stimulates hypothalamic activity and the production of ACTH. It is also very stimulating in general, it can easily raise blood pressure and reduce fasting blood sugar. The dose is 1 to 10 gm per day in an infusion or decoction: 1–6 ml of 1:2 liquid extract. Use the severity of the patient's symptoms and their individual reaction to the herb to determine dose for each case.

American Ginseng *(Panax quinquefolium).* This ginseng is not as hot or stimulating as Chinese ginseng. It has a sedative effect on the central nervous system and has antifatigue qualities as well as antidiuretic action. Dose is 3 to 6 gm of root per day in a decoction.

Korean Ginseng *(Panax ginseng).* This ginseng is essentially the same as Chinese, but is grown in a different region. This gives it a slightly less hot and tonifying nature. A wide dose range, similar to Chinese ginseng, is indicated.

Siberian Ginseng *(Eleuthrococcus senticosus).* This ginseng is not as stimulating as *Panax* and has a general effect on immunity. It also causes a profound increase in stamina. Same dose as *Panax.*

Arctic Root *(Rhodiola rosea).* Excellent tonic, antidepressive, and sexual stimulant, without being overly hot or stimulating. Use in cases where ginseng is too stimulating. Dose: 180 mg, 1 to 2 times per day of tablet form, 2 to 6 ml in liquid form.

Withania *(Withania somnifera;* Ayurvedic name: *ashwagandha).* Called Indian ginseng, it does not have the stimulating properties of ginseng, so using it in the overactive, but debilitated patient may make it more useful than ginseng. Dose: 3–6 gm per day as decoction, 6–12 ml per day of 1:2 liquid extract.

Sarsparilla (*Smilax officinalis*). A cortisol precursor. It may be used as a secondary herb when low cortisol levels are detected. Dose: 1–5 gm per day as decoction, tincture 30 to 40 drops, 3 times a day.

Chinese Medicinals

Because of the variety of manufacturers of the patent formulas that follow, no doses will be given. Each manufacturer will recommend their own dose based on the concentration of the medicinals in its unique formulation.

In adrenal insufficiency, the formulas to consider are as follows:

- Minor Bupleurum Decoction Pills (*Xiao Chai Hu Tang Wan*). Symptoms include alternating chills and fever, nausea, poor appetite, congestion in the lymphatic system, fatigue and/or irritability.
- Tonify Center, Increase Qi Pills (*Bu Zhong Yi Qi Wan*). The symptoms include extreme fatigue, recurrent low-grade fevers, loose stools, cold hands, and feet.
- Adrenosen (Health Concerns Co.). The symptoms include "burn out" with pain, aching, digestive disturbances. Lack of energy with decreased mental acuity. This remedy may be used by those who have come to their present state of health by overuse of stimulants.

Formulas for Cushing's-like symptoms are as follows:

- Six-Flavor Rehmannia Pills (*Liu Wei Di Huang Wan*). The symptoms include mucous membrane dryness, high blood pressure, insomnia, anxiety, dizziness, tinnitus.
- Eight-Flavor Rehmannia Pills (*Zhi Bai Di Huang Wan*). The symptoms include night sweats, hot palms and soles, hot flashes, palpitations, insomnia, anxiety.
- Two Immortals (*Er Xian Tang*; Health Concerns Co.). The symptoms include hot flashes, night sweats, irritability, palpitations, vertigo, insomnia, graying hair, decreased sex drive.

Homeopathy

A search of *Reference Works®* for adrenal yields 55 remedies and 230 references in homeopathic books. The three main polycrest remedies that appear are *Natrum Muriaticum*, *Phosporus*, and *Sepia*. Obviously the other 52 remedies have been found at one time or another to fit adrenal symptoms. Examining the main mental–emotional and some of the physical symptoms of these remedies reveals the relationship to possible adrenal problems.

Natrum Muriaticum (*Nat. Mur.*). One of the main characteristics of this remedy is grief, and a silent grief in particular. *Nat. Mur.* patients can be very serious, depressed, and overly responsible. These characteristics viewed from an adrenal standpoint reveal the symptoms of stress. Much of this stress can be self-induced, like being responsible for others whether they wish it or not. Another self-imposed stress that indicates the need for *Nat. Mur.* is holding on to the grief of a lost love or a death for many years. This kind of mental activity can create an ongoing stress physiology in the body. With a constant stress in the mind, the adrenal glands are called to overwork in a distress, not a eustress, situation.

The person needing *Nat. Mur.* can also dwell on the past and is averse to company. Like many of the mineral salts in homeopathy, this remedy has two sides or is conflicted. Natrum is from the group IA on the periodic table and Muriaticum is the chloride in group VIIA. There is a certain relationship formed by these two elements, the positive and negative ions at once attracting and repulsing one another. One of the main themes of *Nat. Mur.* is relationship. This can mean the patient is overfocused on the making or breaking of a personal relationship. The person may also show great interest in art, music, or literature involving romantic relationships or the breaking of those relationships. The *Nat. Mur.* patient can have many fears and phobias. Examples of these fears are fear of robbers, the dark, storms, insects, germs, and heights. In the Chinese medical paradigm a remedy for the adrenal gland has many fears, because fear is the emotion of the water element, the kidney is the yin organ of that element, and the kidney rules the adrenal gland. The patient who needs *Nat. Mur.* is also claustrophobic, which is interesting for the reasons stated above, but also leads us to think of its use in thyroid conditions, because a thyroid patient commonly has a fear of close spaces. *Nat. Mur.* also has a pronounced craving for salt. Although this is a common symptom for adrenal weakness, it may help to lead to this remedy above others, because the craving can be intense in those who need *Nat. Mur.*

Phosphorus (Phos.). The materia medica of the remedy *Phosphorus* also shows much fear and anxiety; the deeper the condition of the patient, the deeper the fear, even to the point of debilitating phobias. As the pathology of the patient deepens, an exuberant and overly-friendly, even gullible personality changes, to a slow, apathetic, and debilitated person. This symptom is a sign of the adrenal exhaustion taking place. *Phos.* also has a great craving for salt.

Sepia (Sep.). This remedy is the "worn-out washer woman." The *Sep.* patient has worked too long and too hard and is now exhausted. Vithoulkas characterizes this remedy as stasis in all things physical and mental–emotional. However, in the early stages, they may be much more industrious, sensitive, and excitable, somewhat like *Phosphorus*, but later this stasis and exhaustion become the main symptoms. If this kind of reaction is compared to the onset of chronic fatigue syndrome (CFS), believed by many to be adrenal exhaustion, there is a clear similarity in the symptoms of CFS and the above remedies.

Dr. Ramakrishnan finds *Phytolacca* (*Phyto.*) to be the best remedy for adrenal treatment (Ramakrishnan, 2001). Although I can find little reference in the classic literature for its use, his vast clinical experience must be heeded and consideration given to this possible prescription. The *Phyto.* patient can be indifferent to life and have restlessness and prostration.

Gland Cell Therapy

Many companies produce adrenal gland products. From the older texts the daily dose of desiccated adrenal is as follows:

Addison's Disease

- 3 grains, 3 times a day after meals (Sajous, 1922).
- 1–5 grains, 3 times a day (Wolf, 1940).
- Adrenal whole gland ½–2 grains, cortex 2–5 grains, 3–4 times a day (Spring, 1921).
- Adremin 1 tablet, 4 times a day with meals and at bed time (Harrower, 1922).
- Adremin containing 1 grain (60 mg) of adrenal substance (National Formulary VI), the total daily dose is, therefore, 240 mg.
- Adremin also containing endothyrin $\frac{1}{12}$ grain (5 mg), orchic substance 2 grains (120 mg), and calisalin of a sufficient quantity to make up a 5-grain tablet. (Calisalin is a calcium and phosphorus combination used for basic mineral supplementation.) Harrower's product was more akin to Standard Process Company® Symplex M®, without the pituitary substance, than a pure adrenal product.

The Standard Process® line includes three adrenal products, as well as numerous products that contain adrenal in some form to enhance the effect of that supplement.

- Adrenal, Desiccated®. Each tablet supplies 130 mg of bovine adrenal; the usual dose is 1 tablet, 3 times a day.
- Drenatrophin® is strictly a protomorpogen (PMG) product for adrenal support. Each tablet supplies 60 mg (1 grain) bovine adrenal nuclear material. The usual dose is 1 tablet, 3 times a day.
- Drenamin® is a combination product supplying in 3 tablets 50 mg of bovine adrenal and 40 mg bovine adrenal PMG extract. It also contains the ingredients found in Cataplex G®, which is the calming fraction of the B vitamin complex.

Injectable gland cell therapy for adrenal insufficiency has a long history. The first injection of animal material into a human was self-injection by French physician, Brown-Sequard. He used testicular material from a dog and guinea pig as a means of rejuvenation and started the science of endocrinology on its way. These materials are available in most countries outside the United States. The dose of the common dilution 20 mg/ml is, 1 ml by deep intramuscular injection 1 to 2 times per week in severe cases and 1 ml/month in moderate cases.

Nutrition

Vitamins C, E, F, and pantothenic acid. No other gland or tissue has as much ascorbic acid as the adrenal (4.60 ± 0.34 mg per gm of fresh tissue; Bicknell and Prescott, 1953).

Minerals

Phosphorus, calcium, sodium, and tin (Jensen, 1983).

It is interesting to note that the minerals that feed the adrenal glands are also related to the homeopathic remedies useful for the same glands. Phosphorus is on both lists. Sodium is half of the remedy *Nat. Mur.*, which is sodium chloride and sepia comes from cuttlefish ink that is extracted from a cephalopod, and very high in sodium chloride.

An excellent whole food source of these and other minerals is goat whey powder. It is the whey leftover in the cheese-making process and supplies a host of minerals in a whole food, palatable form. A tablespoon once or twice a day is an adequate dose even for severe depletion. Other mineral supplements may be used, but they must be from food sources, not inorganic minerals as are usually sold as high-potency mineral supplements.

Manipulative Therapy

> Relative to their size these glands have a richer innervation than other viscera, their fibers arise from T10, T11, T12, L1.

> (Netter, 1965)

Analysis of the innervation of the adrenals is always a good idea. Simple questioning about the T10 to L1 area may elicit information to warrant a chiropractic evaluation. A palpatory examination might also prove useful. Look for tension, heat, cold, or pain in the tissue adjacent to the spinal levels for adrenal innervation.

For the chiropractor, this examination is a simple matter. For those not trained in manipulation, a referral may be necessary. If any symptoms are elicited on examination or questioning, a referral for examination by someone qualified is important because, from a biomechanical standpoint, if the innervation to the adrenal gland is blocked by subluxation, any other work we may do toward healing the gland will be impeded.

Use the above-mentioned spinal levels for chiropractic or osteopathic manipulation and spondylotherapy.

To use Manaka metronome technique, select kidney meridian, 120 beats per minute, and bladder 112 beats, on any or all of the above-mentioned acupuncture points.

Network therapy, which is not necessarily a chiropractic technique, but is now practiced primarily by chiropractors can help to relieve the stress physiology by regular entrainment.

Neural Therapy

For adrenal insufficiency, inject the sympathetic chain at the upper renal pole (Dosch, 1984). Also, inject intravenously, procaine 1% to help with central regulation of the entire endocrine system (Dosch, 1984). For adrenal overactivity, inject the sympathetic chain at the upper renal pole. The points are the same as those for adrenal insufficiency because neural therapy tends toward regulation, not stimulation or suppression.

The dose is 0.5 to 1 cc per adrenal gland and for the intravenous injection 1 cc in any vein.

Reflexology (a Microsystem)

Reflexology can be used both diagnostically and therapeutically. The adrenal point lies on the bottom of the foot, half way between the transverse lines for the diaphragm and waist, just medial to the tendon flexor hallucis longus (see diagram in microsystems in reflexology chapter).

Color Therapy

Dinshah System

According to Dinshah's method, magenta is used to stimulate the adrenals on areas 4 and 18 (Dinshah, 1939) or scarlet (Dinshah, 1985); to reduce adrenal activity purple is used in the same locations (Dinshah, 1985).

Chakra System

The other methods of color therapy rely on the color/chakra connection. Orange: as a breathing meditation, as ingested color water, as a color selection for clothing. This method balances the second chakra and, therefore, the adrenal gland and the associated spinal levels.

Sound

The tone, according to the chakra system, is E. This tone is delivered to the adrenals by the affected person toning that note with the voice and focusing the intonation on the adrenal gland. Another way to use sound to treat the adrenal gland is to place a tuning fork of E on the back over the adrenal area. To amplify the effect of the tuning fork place a crystal between the fork and the skin. This kind of tonal treatment is another example of the patient being able to perform some of their treatment at home.

Rajan Sankaran relates *Nat. Mur.*, one of the main adrenal homeopathic remedies, to the Indian *Raga Bhairavi*. This raga has the theme of separation or quarrel with a loved one (Sankaran, 1997). This is very similar to the theme of *Nat. Mur.* Some years ago, Sankaran attempted a proving of several ragas of Indian classical music. He did this by having people listen to the music and then note their feelings and sensations, just as Hahnemann advised for ingested homeopathic remedies in a proving. The whole concept of such a complex form of music being proved goes somewhat against the tenets of classical homeopathy, which seeks to prove only a single substance at a time. Perhaps a single tone produced by a tuning fork or tone generator as is suggested for treatment of the adrenal gland according to the chakra system would be more appropriate.

Patient Treatment Protocol

Now is the time to decide on the treatment protocol of integrative endocrinology for each individual patient.

The patients' particular interests should be taken into consideration. Does he or she already do *Qi Gong* or yoga or have some knowledge of color therapy? Is the patient likely to continue on a supplementation routine with gland cell therapy or herbs? Will a change in diet be something that fits easily with the patient's lifestyle? What is the degree of glandular involvement? Will it be necessary to treat with acupuncture or chiropractic weekly for a period of time? Consider these questions and questions related to each of the treatment strategies already mentioned, to determine the extent of the integrative endocrinology program for each individual. The more the program is individualized to the patient's interests, the greater the possibility of compliance and success.

Setting up a program for each person that they will complete is the essence of integrative endocrinology. To make a meaningful change in a person's life by using this method, choose therapies that will be used on a daily basis and not discontinued before the desired healing is manifested in the patient's life. Integrative endocrinology asks the person to incorporate changes in their life that will have an impact on the glandular system and, therefore, have a lasting impact on their health and longevity.

As an example of an integrative endocrinology approach, always start a program with a glandular supplement. The patient will feel better immediately, and using the glands of animals for this purpose is the most direct route to healing. If the person has a severe depletion of the adrenals, begin with whole desiccated adrenal, 1 or 2 tablets, 3 times a day. This is replacement therapy. It is not as invasive and disruptive as the administration of cortisol, but it can have a dramatic and immediate effect. Using desiccated adrenal is similar to using whole thyroid, like Armour thyroid, which is a prescription item for a weak thyroid gland. The difference in using whole adrenal is that it does not contain the large amount of active hormone as the Armour thyroid. This gives the practitioner more latitude in choosing dosage for the purpose of quickly rebuilding the gland without the side effect from the high hormone content. If the problem is not so severe, use Drenatrophin® from Standard Process Company®. This product contains glandular building information in the form of Dr. Lee's protomorphogens. If the patient has the symptoms of being sleepy during the day and waking at night, then use Drenamin® as the first prescription. This product contains adrenal protomorhogen and whole adrenal, both in small amounts, and the calming portion of the B complex vitamins.

Next, depending on the severity of the case, select a herb from the list provided. If the case has many mental–emotional components, not just physical weakness, choose a homeopathic remedy to complete the internal medicine–prescribing portion of the case.

Give this internal regimen for 3 to 6 months, then evaluate for any changes that need to be made on the basis of patients' progress. If healing has not proceeded, next choose among acupuncture, neural therapy, chiropractic, and massage. You may want to add additional therapies sooner, depending on your personal practice and the severity of the case. The practitioner's personal expertise will determine where to turn first. The reasons for selection of one technique over another are given in the individual therapy chapters.

Recommending self-help techniques to enhance the clinical work may be of great help to improve the treatment. It is often very helpful to teach a few acupuncture points for acupressure. It is a good idea to provide a diagram for the patient to aid his or her memory. Teaching the adrenal reflexology point for self-massage is also an excellent way to allow the patient to participate in their own treatment. Music, color meditations, or color water are all things the patient can do at home. Many patients are very appreciative when they are included in the therapy. Other patients just want the treatment handled for them. The more integrative the approach, the better chance the person has to overcome their glandular difficulties.

Some Case Histories

The following are three short, anecdotal stories from the author's practice to show how common occurrences in daily practice can be endocrine related. These cases require holistic thinking through the prism of endocrinology.

A patient was sent to Dr. Beans after consultation with two medical doctors. The patient was a 54-year-old female, somewhat over weight, and reporting stress and exhaustion. She also presented with some unusual symptoms, including a feeling of extreme heat, like being roasted from the inside and very intolerant of heat. She was occasionally incontinent of urine, especially when coughing or laughing. She had a complete blood workup that revealed little of diagnostic value to the MDs. A cortisol level had been drawn and was slightly inside the low-normal range. The case appeared to be one of adrenal fatigue with low-normal lab values. However, on closer inspection, the time of the lab test was 7:40 a.m. The patient lived 40 miles from the hospital. The circadian rhythm of cortisol was not taken into consideration and the stress of the drive. The patient was treated with desiccated adrenal one TID and the homeopathic remedy causticum 30c. This treatment gave quick and sure results. The symptoms fit well with the use of *Causticum* as the remedy. The main point of interest is the patient showed clear symptoms of adrenal exhaustion, but the adrenal gland was not considered because the lab repot showed the cortisol level to be in the normal range without consideration of the circadian rhythm.

Dr. Beans was called by an old college friend to see her mother who was recently hospitalized for 3 days, with unexplained symptoms. The patient had weakness, weight gain, but only in the central part of the body, while the arms and legs remained thin. She had noticeable facial hair and definite striations on the abdomen. This woman had been seeking medical care for these symptoms for 3 years. In less than 1 minute there were two glaringly apparent questions: Was this a cortisol-secreting adrenal tumor creating Cushing's syndrome? Or an ACTH-secreting pituitary tumor creating Cushing's disease? These questions were easily answered by an abdominal ultrasound that showed a clear adrenal tumor. Unfortunately the patient died before any therapy could be initiated. Clearly, this was a case for surgery followed by a program of integrative endocrinology.

Case three is a 22-year-old actress and recently certified Pilates teacher. As she began teaching Pilates exercise classes she lost 20 pounds. She is now in the best physical shape of her life. During this same time, she developed acne. She has visited many doctors, including a dermatologist, without resolving the problem. I believe the decrease in fat led to a decrease in production and conversion of estrogens causing the adrenal glands to increase production of DHEA. This could easily be the cause of the recent onset of acne. For doctors who use hormone replacement, a common side effect of too much DHEA is acne. Also, the adrenal glands interpret the sudden increase in physical activity as stress and produce more cortisol and DHEA to compensate.

These cases demonstrate the need to not dismiss any symptom and to link the available symptoms together for a unified diagnosis.

14 Thyroid Gland

Function and Biochemistry

Location: At the neck, below the cricoid cartilage of the trachea, a small band or isthmus, joins two lobes on either side of the neck.
Size: The lobes are 4 cm long and 2 to 2.5 cm wide. The isthmus is 2 cm high, 2 cm wide, and 0.5 cm thick.
Weight: 15 to 20 gm.
Structure: Homogeneous tissue.

Hormones Produced

The thyroid gland makes two hormones. About 80% of hormone production is T4 or thyroxin and 20% is T3 or triiodothyronine. The storage and transport form of thyroid hormone is T4. The peripheral tissues convert T4 to T3. T3 is the active form of thyroid hormone so T4 converts to T3 before it can act on the cells of the body. The conversion process is called deiodination. One of the iodine molecules is broken off making a hormone with three iodine molecules instead of four. Unlike the other endocrine glands, the thyroid stores a reserve of thyroid hormone enough to create a euthyroid state for 50 days (Williams, 2003).

Signs and Symptoms of Disorder or Dysfunction

Part of the physical examination of a thyroid patient includes a through palpation of the thyroid gland to detect tissue abnormalities. Detecting nodules may be an indication for thyroid ultrasound. These ultrasounds are increasingly available. However, with the increase in ultrasound, there is an increase in the detection of benign thyroid nodules that would not have been discovered without it. The question then arises, is investigation with ultrasound necessary for every nodule detected by palpation? Further, should every nodule seen on ultrasound receive a biopsy? These questions have yet to be answered, but keep them in mind when investigating the thyroid.

Hyperthyroidism is an increased function of the gland. A characteristic symptom is increased heart rate of over 100 beats per minute. In the case of a severely overactive gland, the heart rate can be so fast that it is nearly impossible to count. Other symptoms include weight loss, aversion to heat, or sunlight.

The overproduction or overadministration of thyroid hormone can cause severe trembling. This overactivity can stem from an unknown cause, autoimmunity, a tumor, or may be iatrogenic. Interferon, administered as a treatment for hepatitis C can cause a very severe form of hyperthyroidism.

The ordinary medical solution for an overactive thyroid is to ablate the gland with radioactive iodine or to surgically remove the gland and replace its function with the administration of a synthetic hormone. There are also drugs to slow the function of the gland.

In integrative endocrinology, many of our treatment strategies are effective for a hyperthyroid condition. If the condition is autoimmune then the use of an oral tolerance material is probably the best choice, along with providing the gland with nutritional material to rebuild structure and function. Tracking the success of this treatment is easy by following the thyroid autoantibodies on a blood test.

Hypothyroidism is the underfunction of the thyroid gland. Some authorities believe that as many as 80% of people aged over 40 years have some mild form of hypothyroid problem. The symptoms of low thyroid function are feeling cold, being overweight with an inability to lose weight, fatigue, slow pulse, dry skin and hair, and Queen Anne's sign that is a thinning of the outer third of the eyebrows.

Why is the thyroid gland so affected in the world today? Many believe it is the competition for iodine receptor sites in the thyroid gland by the other halogens, that is, the other elements in Group VIIa on the periodic table of the elements.

The mechanism behind "halogen displacement" was probably best described by D.C. Jarvis MD who wrote:

> The clinical activity of any one of these four halogens is in inverse proportion to its atomic weight. This means that any one of the four can displace the element with a higher atomic weight, but cannot displace an element with a lower atomic weight. For example, fluorine can displace chlorine, bromine, and iodine because fluorine has a lower atomic weight than the other three. Similarly, chlorine can displace bromine and iodine because they both have a higher atomic weight. Likewise, bromine can displace iodine from the body because iodine has a higher atomic weight. But a reverse order is not possible. A knowledge of this well-known chemical law brings us to a consideration of the addition

of chlorine to our drinking water as a purifying agent. We secure a drinking water that is harmful to the body not because of its harmful germ content but because the chlorine content now causes the body to lose the much-needed iodine.

(Jarvis, 1958)

There is now considerable experimentation taking place with dramatically increased iodine supplementation with some authorities using from 12.5 to 50 mg per day in supplemental iodine. One of the positive effects of this dramatic increase in the administration of iodine above the recommended daily allowance from the United States Department of Agriculture is the displacement seems to be reversible, that is, with high doses of iodine, the thyroid begins to clear other halogens like fluorine and bromine.

One of the arguments against such high doses of dietary iodine is the Wolff–Chiakoff effect. There is suppression of thyroid production of T4 with the administering of increasing doses of iodine. This seems to be true when iodine is used in these high doses initially, which means that if a patient is in a hyperthyroid state and immediate suppression of T4 is needed for a short time this high-dose iodine method can be used. However, in as little as 2 weeks the body overcomes the effect of T4 suppression and production of thyroid hormones returns to normal (Abraham, 2005).

Testing Function

Broda Barnes, in his book *Hypothyroidism: The unsuspected illness*, reveals a simple test for thyroid function. The patient takes his or her axillary temperature every morning before rising. Normal temperature upon waking and before any movement is between 97.8 F and 98.2 F. An axillary temperature below 97.8 F indicates a low-functioning thyroid and a temperature above 98.2 F can indicate an overfunction of the thyroid.

Testing iodine is a good idea because it is so necessary to thyroid function. The patient can perform a simple test at home. Iodine is painted on the skin in a 3-inch square on the lower abdomen, the inner thigh, or the inner arm. Begin this test before bed. In the morning, the color is noted. If the patch looks the same in the morning as it did in the evening, then no iodine deficiency exists. If the skin shows no iodine staining then the deficiency is severe. This test gives an indirect measure of the amount of iodine circulating in that person.

There are many laboratory tests for thyroid function. Each of these tests detects a different aspect of thyroid function or of the effect of thyroid hormones on other organs and tissues. The two main tests are the thyroid stimulating hormone (TSH) and the free T4 (thyroxin). These two tests constitute the ordinary medical screening for thyroid disorders. This author also tests free T3 on initial screening. T3 is the active form of thyroid hormone. A comparison between T4 and T3 allows the practitioner to see how much of the transport form is in the blood stream and how much has been converted for use.

Other important tests are for thyroid autoantibodies. These tests detect antibodies to thyroid peroxidase and thyroglobulin. Occurring usually after a thyroid injury, these test help to diagnose Hashimoto's thyroiditis.

Therapy

Acupuncture

- St-10 (*Shui tu,* Water Prominence) 3 cun superior to the median end of the clavicle at the anterior border of the sternocleidomastoid muscle.

For Hypothyroid Add

- TW-3 (*Zhong Zhu,* Central Islet) dorsum of the hand between the fourth and fifth metacarpal bones just proximal to the metacarpalphalageal joint.
- LI-4 (*He Gu,* Joining Valley) hold the thumb and forefinger together; the point is at the highest point of the first interosseous muscle.

For Hyperthyroid Add

- St-44 (*Nei Ting,* Inner Courtyard) just proximal to the web margin between the second and third toe.
- LV-3 (*Tai Chong,* Great Rushing) top of the foot in the hollow distal to the junction of the first and second metatarsal bones. Usually the dorsalis pedis artery can be felt pulsing.

Homeopathy

Iodum (*Iod.*). This remedy is iodine in homeopathic form. Its symptoms are those of hyperthyroidism. Restless, trembling, hot, irritable. Hungry with weight loss.

Calcarea Carbonica (*Calc. Carb.*) this remedy is the calcium from the center layer of an oyster shell. *Calc. Carb.* is the perfect picture of hypothyroidism: overweight, cold, slow.

Sepia (*Sep.*) is the ink from the cuttlefish. The symptoms are that of the worn-out washerwoman: exhausted, overweight, irritable.

Natrum Muriaticum (*Nat. Mur.*) is sodium chloride and has a great affinity for the thyroid gland. The person needing *Nat. Mur.* is emotionally reserved, very responsible, and affected by grief, even grief long past.

Gland Cell Therapy

The main product used by ordinary medicine is whole, desiccated thyroid gland of porcine origin. According to Western medical texts, Murray in Scotland first used whole sheep thyroid gland for the treatment of myxedema in 1891.

Using whole thyroid gland in this form requires a prescription; consequently, many natural health care providers do not have access to this therapy.

As is often the case with Western medicine, this "original thought" was not original at all. More than 800 years earlier, Sun Su Mo in his *Thousand Golden Prescriptions* described the use of whole sheep thyroid gland for use in goiter and hypothyroidism. This product is often referred to as "Armour thyroid" because the Armour meat packing company was one of the last producers of whole thyroid for medical use. In fact, in older materia medicas, there were many companies making thyroid. The use of whole thyroid approximates the use of synthetic T4 (levothyroxin).

The synthetic form of T4 is manufactured in a variety of specific microgram strengths. Measurement of the natural whole gland equivalent is by weight of the glandular material, not hormone content. Much of the controversy in using whole gland thyroid instead of its synthetic counterpart centers on the erroneous idea that, because the synthetic hormone is precisely measured, the dose is more accurate. This commonly used argument is false.

The US Pharmacopoeia requires synthetic thyroid hormone to be only 90% to 110% of the amount stated on the label. In addition, there is a wide range of absorbability depending on foods eaten and on the ability of the small intestine to absorb the hormone. Administration of thyroid hormone, as with any other hormone, suppresses secretion of thyroid hormone from the gland by suppressing the secretion of thyroid-stimulating hormone (TSH) from the pituitary (PDR 1513). This suppression changes the balance between the TSH and T4.

Absorption varies from 48 to 80% of the administered dose (PDR 1513).

If you give 100 µg of synthetic T4 and it is only 90% of what was on the label and only 48% is absorbed; then the dose the patient gets is 43.2 µg. This is not an exact science.

Many companies produce thyroid gland cell products without thyroxin. Great success comes when using these products. It is not necessary to have high hormone content or any hormone content at all, to be effective. In fact, in the case of using a thyroid gland cell product, it is better to have the thyroxin removed. Because of removal of the thyroxin, the practitioner is free to use as much gland cell product as is necessary without the side effect of the hormone. This might be necessary in the case of Hashimoto's thyroiditis with very high autoantibodies. For oral tolerance to be effective, it is sometimes necessary to use a very large dose to calm the autoimmune attack.

In addition, products without added synthetic vitamins or minerals are best because the practitioner can easily individualize supplementation in addition to the gland. If there are additives, the practitioner must use the predetermined formulation. This formulation does not allow the practitioner to use as much or as little thyroid gland as needed and independently decide on other nutrients.

- Oral $\frac{1}{12}$ to 1 gr three times a day (Sajous, 1922).
- Oral, 19 products from $\frac{1}{10}$ to 5 gm; injectable, four products ranging from $\frac{1}{100}$ to 5 gm, 1 to 3 times a day (Wolf, 1940).
- Oral, begin with 0.25 gm and increase as needed (Spring, 1921).
- Oral, $\frac{1}{10}$ to 1 gm, 3 times a day (Harrower, 1922).

The Standard Process® product Thytrophin® is excellent for cases of hypothyroid or hyperthyroid. It is particularly useful in cases of autoimmune thyroiditis because it is a protomorphogen or PMG product.

Manipulative Therapy

Use spinal-level C6 and C7 for chiropractic or osteopathic manipulation and spondylotherapy.

To use Manaka metronome technique select triple-burner meridian, 152 beats per minute and stomach 132 beats, on any or all of the above-mentioned acupuncture points.

Western Herbal Medicine

- Poke root (*Phytolacca decandra*), especially for goiter (Hutchens, 1973).
- Seaweeds like kelp, dulse, hiziki, and nori.
- Cocoa (*Theobroma cacao*) thyroid regulator (PDR Herbs, 211).
- Bugleweed (*Lycopus virginicus*).

Neural Therapy

Inject directly into the lobes of the thyroid gland. The patient should be positioned on the back and asked to swallow to locate the gland precisely.

Color Therapy

Chakra System

Blue on the throat area.

Dinshah System

- Thyroid underactivity: orange 7 to 15, and lemon, systemic front
- Hyperthyroid: lemon 22, and indigo systemic front, green on #1
- Thyroiditis: green systemic front, blue on #3.

Chinese Medicinals

- Neck Mass Pills (*Yi Kang Wan*). For symptoms of hyperthyroid, 3 to 4 pills, 3 times a day.
- Sargassum Teapills (*Hai Zao Wan*). For use in swellings especially goiter, 8 to 12 pills, 3 times a day. Only one seaweed is contained in this remedy.
- Haiodin (*Hai Zao Wan*). Also for goiter, 2 pills, 3 times a day. This remedy contains two kinds of seaweed.

Hypothyroid Herbs

- *Fu Zi* (*Radix aconiti lateralis praeparata*). 3 to 15 gm.
- *Kun Bu* (*Thallus laminariae seu eckloniae*). 10 to15 gm.
- *Rou Gui* (*Cortex cinnamomi*). 2 to 5 gm.

Sound

The tone for thyroid is G.

Dietary Considerations

The thyroid requires at least 150 µg of iodine per day. In the United States, iodine intake is decreasing because of lower salt intake. In addition, in the late 1960s, the iodine in bread was replaced by bromine because it was thought that Americans were getting too much dietary iodine. Increasing the amount of iodine can inhibit the release of T4 (*Williams Textbook of Endocrinology*, 2003: 336). This is the Wolff–Chaikoff effect. The body overcomes or escapes from this suppressive effect of iodine even in high doses. High iodine intake can, in rare cases, lead to hyperthyroidism. This is the Jod–Basedow effect.

On the periodic table of the elements, Group VIIa contains fluorine, chlorine, bromine, iodine, and astatine. Iodine is the primary nutrient for the thyroid gland. It is essential because it is a major component of thyroid hormones T4 and T3. If other elements in the same group are ingested, for instance, fluorine in water or toothpaste, this can interfere with the uptake of iodine by the thyroid. Blocked iodine uptake creates a condition of hypofunction of the thyroid.

Some Case Notes

For a female initially aged 62.

May 2003

TSH 8.56 (0.40–7.00), free T4 0.7 (0.7–2.2), free T3 96 (70–180)

Even though the thyroid hormone values were still in range, the TSH was elevated, and most important, this woman was having clear symptoms of hypothyroid. She experienced dry skin, hair loss, fatigue, and she was cold all the time.

Antithyroglobulin and antiperoxidase antibodies were both tested on the initial screening and were not present. These symptoms and lab tests confirm that this is a case of simple hypothyroidism.

The patient had acupuncture once a month and Thytrophin PMG® 1 tablet, 3 times a day. The thyroxin (T4) is removed from the thyroid gland material. In this case, in contrast with a case of using levothyroxin, the lowering of TSH is not due to suppression from exogenous T4 but a repair of the thyroid gland so it can produce its own hormone. This is also a protomorphogen product, which means it contains only the nuclear material from the thyroid cells.

There are two possible actions for the thyroid gland material. Either the gland material is acting as a decoy (oral tolerance) for the immune system, giving the thyroid a chance to repair while the immune system attacks the oral gland material in the gut or the material is acting as nourishment for the gland so it can rebuild healthy tissue. In this case, the latter explanation is the most likely because no autoimmune reaction was shown on blood tests.

November 2003

TSH 4.74 (0.40–7.00), Free T4 0.9 (0.7–2.2), T3 133 (70–180)

Discontinuing the acupuncture treatment, the patient continued on Thytrophin.

May 2004

TSH 4.46 (0.40–7.00), Free T4 1.04 (0.70–2.2), T3 163 (70–180)

The patient is free of her previous symptoms and is no longer taking thytrophin.

15 Hypothalamus Gland

Function and Biochemistry

The hypothalamus allows us to maintain homeostasis. It monitors the endocrine system and coordinates autonomic and behavioral responses. It receives information from outside the body in the form of light, temperature, pain, and odors. It also receives information from the internal body environment like blood pressure, blood glucose, and hormone levels.

Location: Inside the cranium, just above the pituitary gland.
Size: A few cubic centimeters, about the size of an almond.
Weight: 1/300 of the total brain weight.
Structure: Three separate structures compose the hypothalamus:

* Pars nervosa
* Infundibular stalk
* Median eminence.

The effects produced by different areas further divide the hypothalamus. As many as 12 separate and distinct areas of influence exist in this very small gland.

Hormones Produced

The hormones produced and secreted by the hypothalamus go directly to the pituitary through the portal vessels of the pituitary stalk. These hormones have a stimulating or inhibiting effect on pituitary hormone production. The hypothalamus is where the nervous system ultimately connects to the endocrine system.

Hormones are secreted by two types of neurons projecting to the external zone of the median eminence.

Peptide Neurons

- Thyrotropin-releasing hormone (TRH), the first of the releasing hormones, discovered in 1970. The hormone stimulates the pituitary to secrete thyroid-stimulating hormone (TSH). It is a potent releaser of prolactin (PRL) and can also release corticotropin (ACTH) and growth hormone (HGH).
- Corticotropin-releasing hormone (CRH) stimulates release of adrenocorticotropic hormone (ACTH).
- Luteinizing hormone-releasing hormone (LHRH) stimulates release of LH.

Neurons Containing Bioamines

- Dopamine is the primary prolactin inhibiting factor (PIF).
- Serotonin is synthesized from tryptophan and is the precursor of melatonin. It is synthesized in many tissues. It is a neurotransmitter, inhibits gastric secretions, and it stimulates smooth muscle.

Other

- Gonadotropin-releasing hormone (GnRH) stimulates secretion of follicle stimulating hormone (FSH) and luteinizing hormone (LH).
- Somatostatin inhibits the release of growth hormone.
- Vasopressin (AVP) also called antidiuretic hormone (ADH) is responsible for water balance.
- Oxytocin stimulates uterine contraction and milk letdown.

Signs and Symptoms of Disorder or Dysfunction

The main signs and symptoms of disorders of the hypothalamus are not directly observable. They are detected as signs of the dysfunction of end glands become apparent. As an example, the signs and symptoms of hypothyroidism may be your first clue to the decreased release of thyrotrophin-releasing hormone (TRH). In addition, a decrease in thyroid-stimulating hormone (TSH) or the thyroid hormones T4 or T3 may indicate decreased TRH. The hypothalamus is not the most likely cause of hypothyroidism, but should be considered if ordinary measures are not helping the condition. An extreme increase in urination may be the clue to a decrease in Vasopressin, the cause of diabetes insipidus.

In conditions like post-traumatic stress disorder, the author treats the entire hypothalamus–pituitary–adrenal axis; this seems to speed recovery though there is no way to prove direct involvement of the hypothalamus.

Testing Function

Bedside diagnosis of hypothalamic disorders is imprecise at best. However, many changes in easily observable symptoms may help point to hypothalamic disorders. These symptoms include changes in temperature regulation, appetite and thirst disorders, obesity, increased urination, sleep disorders, and autonomic or behavioral changes. Many of the hypothalamic hormones are testable by blood, urine, or saliva if a defined number is required for a definitive diagnosis. This author only uses direct testing of the hypothalamus if therapy is not having a positive result.

Therapy

Acupuncture

- GV-20 (*Bai Hui*, Hundred Meetings) on the midline at the vertex of the head if a line is drawn between the tops of the ears.
- LI-4 (*He Gu*, Joining Valley). Hold the thumb and forefinger together; the point is at the highest point of the first interosseous muscle.
- M-HN-3 (*Yin Tang*, Hall of Impression) at the midpoint between the eyebrows.
- K-7 (*Fu Liu*, Returning Current) 2 cun above the medial maleolus at the anterior border of the Achilles tendon.
- K-1 (*Yong Quan*, Gushing Spring) on the bottom of the foot, between the second and third metatarsal bones about one-third the distance from the base of the second toe to the heel.
- TW-20 (*Jiao Sun*, Minute Angle) on the side of the head directly level with the top of the ear.

Homeopathy

The French method explained in the homeopathy chapter is the best approach to known hypothalamus disorders. In the computer program *Reference Works®* there are 75 references and 20 remedies. These remedies are difficult to define in relation to the hypothalamus, as there are only vague references to the gland. There is no discussion of specific functional alterations in the hypothalamus.

Treating the hypothalamus is an opportunity to combine two levels of therapy. If you are certain of the involvement of the hypothalamus in a disease process such as post-traumatic stress disorder (see adrenal chapter on PTSD), you may want to create your own homeopathic remedy from the available gland cell therapy remedies as explained in the homeopathic chapter. You will then be giving the gland in its material dose and the gland in homeopathic form. There may be some benefit to using the same material in glandular and homeopathic preparations. This benefit is giving the same informational signal to the gland in material as well as potentized form. Homeopathic hypothalamus is also available in low potencies from many pharmacies to treat following the French method.

Gland Cell Therapy

The hypothalamus is not mentioned in the pre-1940s books selected to demonstrate dose levels of glandular material in other chapters; therefore, only modern doses can be demonstrated.

Standard Process® has two hypothalamus products:

- Hypothalmex® is a whole gland product supplying 140mg of bovine hypothalamus per tablet.
- Hypothalamus PMG® is a protomorphogen product supplying 140mg of bovine hypothalamus nucleoproteins per tablet.

It has been this author's practice to use only one tablet per day of either of these products. Even in severe cases of PTSD, this dose seems adequate to help the symptoms of paranoia and agoraphobia that develop in the later stages.

Manipulative Therapy

Use spinal-level C1 for chiropractic or osteopathic manipulation and spondylotherapy.

To use Manaka metronome technique, select kidney meridian, 120 beats per minute, on any or all of the above-mentioned acupuncture points.

Western Herbal Medicine

Specific herbs are not listed for the hypothalamus; however, the adaptogenic herbs like the ginsengs, ashwaganda, and maca root may be of possible use.

Neural Therapy

The exact crown of the head, 0.25 to 0.50 c.

Color Therapy

Chakra System

Violet on the crown of the head.

Dinshah System

Blue as a pineal stimulant, area 1 or green as a pituitary stimulant and equilibrator, and area 1. There is no reference in the texts.

Sound

Chakra sound B.

A Case Study

One of the most interesting cases of successful treatment of the hypothalamus is the case of the author's dog. The dog—we will call her A for anonymity—was a Samoyed retriever cross. At some time around the middle of her 15-year life, she must have been shot at. In Montana, this is a common occurrence because according to Montana law a dog may be killed if it is seen chasing livestock. Her personality changed from being unafraid of a pistol shot nearby to being terrified by distant gunfire and all forms of electrical storm activity. These fears caused such anxiety reactions that she was inconsolable and at times uncontrollable. During a thunderstorm, she would run away for hours. When tied to a nearby tree, she nearly hung herself by repeatedly jumping a fence during storm activity.

The diagnosis was simple: post-traumatic stress disorder (PTSD). A past trauma had effected the endocrine system in such a way that similar events in the present brought back the same emotional and physiologic stress as had occurred with the original stress. This is a situation not unlike two Vietnam veterans 30 years after the war, walking along a country road and ducking as a helicopter flies overhead. However, A's symptoms were much more dramatic.

Long before a thunderstorm arrived, she would jump on the side of the house to come in. Fireworks anywhere in the neighborhood sparked disaster. One New Years' Eve, when confined to the laundry room during a fireworks display next door, she tore through the water hose for the washing machine and flooded the house.

Every treatment was tried: acupuncture, every homeopathic remedy possible, every suggested drug like tranquilizers, benzodiazepines, dramamine, benadryl. We also tried eye movement desensitization and reprocessing (EMDR); none of these treatments was helpful in reducing her fear reaction.

The question came to mind, "where is the seat of fear?" The gland where fear arises is the adrenal. This is what produces the fight or flight reaction. These are A's symptoms. However, if you think about it, the brain and nervous system are the beginning of the fear reaction. The nervous system connects to the hypothalamus and pituitary to stimulate the adrenaline reaction.

I gave the dog Standard Process® Hypothalmex®, one tablet per day and within 3 to 4 months she began to respond to the therapy as she had not in years of trying other treatment methods. Now she receives the remedy once a month and continues to be symptom free.

If there is high-powered rifle fire at our next door neighbor's house, the dog still has some mild anxiety but, no longer to thunderstorms.

This is the perfect case of PTSD solved with one simple remedial action. This same approach has been used on several veterans of the Vietnam War. Many years after the trauma of war, the symptoms of adrenal exhaustion may manifest. The adrenal gland may take time to wear down to the point where the symptoms are noticeable. As the adrenal gland begins to underfunction, the pituitary and hypothalamus begin to increase function. This is when the agoraphobia and paranoia begin.

Summary

The hypothalamus is such a complex gland that it is hard to observe individual hormonal malfunctions. For example, if the hypothalamus produces less CRH than necessary, it is hard to prescribe for that one imbalance. A direct approach for treating the whole gland is the most useful. The integrative approach might include acupuncture, neural therapy, and gland or sarcode therapy. To continue with a truly integrative solution, treating the imbalance caused by the hypothalamus malfunction is necessary. The thorough practitioner, faced with a case of PTSD, may choose to treat the obvious adrenal exhaustion and then perhaps the not-so-obvious effects on the pituitary and hypothalamus.

The hypothalamus is truly the master gland. It receives neural and hormonal signals from all parts of the body. After interpreting these signals, the gland then releases the hormones that ultimately control the secretions of the pituitary.

16 Pituitary Gland

Function and Biochemistry

The pituitary gland has two separate and distinct lobes. The posterior lobe is a reservoir for antidiuretic hormone (ADH) produced in the hypothalamus and it produces oxytocin. The anterior lobe produces the six hormones responsible for regulating most of the major functions of the endocrine system by negative feedback with the other glands.

Location: In the cranium. Protected by a small bony cup called the sella turcica.
Size: Round, about the size of a garden pea.
Weight: 600 mg.

Hormones Produced

- Prolactin (PRL)
- Growth hormone (HGH) human growth hormone
- Adrenocorticotropic hormone (ACTH)
- Luteinizing hormone (LH)
- Follicle-stimulating hormone (FSH)
- Thyroid-stimulating hormone (TSH)
- Antidiuretic hormone (ADH) or antivasopressin hormone (AVP) store and releases only
- Oxytocin.

Function of Hormones

Prolactin (PRL), as the name implies, is responsible for milk production. Overproduction of PRL, called hyperprolactinemia, is usually caused by a tumor or prolactinoma and is a medical (drug) or surgical problem if it is not treated with integrative techniques soon enough. In the normal pituitary, the ratio of HGH cells to PRL cells is 10:1. The hormone content of the gland is about 100 µg. During pregnancy and lactation, the PRL cells may become 70% of the gland.

Growth hormone (GH) or (HGH) is responsible for overall growth by its action on insulin-like growth factor-1 (IGF-1). It is used for the treatment of idiopathic short stature in children. In adults, GH helps maintain primary tissues like muscle, skin, and bone.

Adrenocorticotropic hormone (ACTH) is secreted in a circadian rhythm with the high point starting at 3 a.m. to 7 a.m. and the low point from 11 p.m. to 3 a.m. Within this circadian cycle, there are also 40 pulses per 24 hours. Giving corticosteroids suppresses this pattern. ACTH is responsible for the functions, size, and structure of the adrenal cortex.

Luteinizing hormone (LH) and follicle-stimulating hormone (FSH) are gonadotrophic hormones. The cells responsible for their production occupy about 10% to 15% of the anterior pituitary.

Interaction with Other Glands

PRL is under tonic inhibitory control of the hypothalamus. This means that cutting the stalk between the hypothalamus and pituitary, hyperprolactinemia is one result. The main hormone creating this control of PRL is dopamine. Many hormones can stimulate the overproduction of PRL. Some examples are estrogens, thyroid-releasing hormone (TRH), serotonin, and its precursors like tryptophan or 5-HTP. In addition, the serotonin reuptake inhibitors (Prozac® etc.), which cause an increase in serum levels of serotonin, can cause an increase in PRL.

Growth hormone stimulates insulin-like growth factor 1 (IGF-1). The IGF-1 then exerts a negative feedback with the hypothalamus and pituitary, decreasing the secretion of GH. The hypothalamus secretes growth hormone–releasing hormone (GHRH) and somatotropin release–inhibiting factor (SRIF) independently. These two hormones interact to produce the pulsatile release of GH from the pituitary. The synthesis of GH is also affected by somatostatin, ghrelin, thyroid hormone, and glucocorticoids.

ACTH is the middle hormone in the hypothalamus–pituitary–adrenal (HPA) axis. During any stress response corticotropin–releasing hormone (CRH) from the hypothalamus stimulates ACTH. This causes an increase in secretion of ACTH that stimulates release of adrenal hormones, especially cortisol.

Luteinizing hormone (LH) in females is responsible for androgen hormone production and oocyte maturation. In males, LH is responsible for testicular synthesis of testosterone.

Follicle-stimulating hormone (FSH) in females regulates ovarian estrogen production. In males, it probably regulates sperm development.

The cells producing LH and FSH are about 10% to 15% of the anterior pituitary cells.

Signs and Symptoms of Disorder or Dysfunction

Signs of an increase of PRL include lactation and infertility. If the patient has headaches or visual disturbance, this is a sign of advanced disease and requires referral to a clinical endocrinologist. In any pituitary problem when these signs are present, it is an indication of a tumor that is pressing on the optic chiasm or other structure near the pituitary. This requires immediate regular medical attention.

As with the hypothalamus, the terminal endocrine gland is usually seen as the presenting problem. If therapy is not having the expected result or the problem is chronic, you may want to consider pituitary therapy.

Testing Function

Tests for all the pituitary hormones are available with clinical laboratory blood tests. Many of these tests are very common. Measuring TSH to assess thyroid function or LH and FSH for fertility or menopause is routine. The pituitary hormones also occur in the urine. The advantage to urinary testing is that the measurement is for 24 hours, so you may assess the total function of the gland, not just the amount of hormone in the blood stream at the time of the draw.

Therapy

Acupuncture

- EM-3 (*Yin Tang*, Hall of Impression) midpoint between the eyebrows.
- GV-20 (*Bai Hui*, Hundred Meetings) on the midline at the vertex of the head. It is interesting that the Chinese acupuncturists felt that this one point treated one hundred diseases. Did they understand the connection with the pituitary?

Homeopathy

A total of 247 references and 73 remedies occur in *Reference Works®*. Because of its complex function, selecting a homeopathic remedy based only on hypo- or hyper-pituitarism is nearly impossible. Many of the remedies listed in *Reference Works®* relate to the pituitary. As examples, both cortisol and folliculinum are mentioned. Both of these remedies are part of an axis that includes the pituitary, but they are not indicated for direct treatment of pituitary disorders. The remedies themselves do not necessarily directly affect the pituitary.

The pituitary is another example of a good place to use the French method in conjunction with other therapies. You may want to reserve the use of homeopathy to cases where the first line methods you choose are not effective enough. A homeopathic remedy prescribed by the French method and perhaps even handmade from the gland cell therapy product you are using may be just the thing to move a case forward.

Gland Cell Therapy

* Oral: 3 to 5 grains, 3 times a day (Sajous, 1922).
* Oral: ½ to 5 grains, 3 times a day; injectable: 0.5 to 1cc, 3 times a week (Wolf, 1940).
* Oral: posterior pituitary, ¼ to 1 grain, 3 to 4 times a day; anterior pituitary, 1 to 4 grains, 3 to 4 times a day (Spring, 1921).
* Oral: 5 to 30 grains per day; injectable: 1 to 2 cc, once a day (Harrower, 1922).
* Standard Process Pituitrophin PMG®, oral: 45 mg, 3 times a day.

Manipulative Therapy

Spinal-level C1 for chiropractic, osteopathic, and spondylotherapy applications.

For Manaka, remember that in Oriental medicine the kidney meridian rules the brain, so use 120 beats per minute tapping over C1.

Western Herbal Medicine

As with the hypothalamus, little research exists on specific herbs for the pituitary. The adaptogens are useful if you are unable to get adequate results from a combination of other therapies. Another reason to use adaptogenic herbs is in the case of a vegetarian who will not take an animal product such as pituitary substance.

Alfalfa (*Medicago sativa*) has prolactin-inhibiting effects.

Neural Therapy

The point is in the center of the forehead. Use 0.25 to 0.50 cc.

Color Therapy

Chakra System

Indigo in the middle of the forehead.

Dinshah System

* Acromegaly: lemon systemic front, green and indigo on #1.
* Hypopituitarism: green on #1.

- Diabetes insipitus: lemon systemic front, green on #1, orange on #3, indigo on # 1–15 if cerebral tumor, magenta on #18.
- Secondary adrenal insufficiency: lemon systemic back, green on #1, indigo on 1 to 15 if tumor.

Chinese Medicinals

- Radix Rehmanniae (*Sheng Di Huang*). 10 to 30 gm in decoction.
- Radix Anemarrhenae (*Zhi Mu*).
- Radix Glycyrrhizae (*Gan Cao*).
- Radix Ginseng (*Ren Shen*). Good in combination with Gan Cao.
- Herba Cistanches (*Rou Cong Rong*).
- Radix Morindae Officinalis (*Ba Ji Tian*).

Sound

Chakra system tone A. If you are toning or using a tuning fork or tone generator look at the diagram of the location of the pituitary and focus on this area with the tone.

17 Pineal Gland

Function and Biochemistry

The pineal gland has the appearance of pinecone. This is the origin of the name.

The pineal produces melatonin. This is the sleep hormone. Some people believe that the pineal deteriorates and calcifies with age and this is what leads to sleep disturbances in the elderly.

Location: In the midline of the brain, posterior to the pituitary.
Size: 8 mm long
Weight: 100 to 200 mg.
Structure: Pinealocytes, these cells are primitive photoreceptive cells and interstitial or glial cells.

Hormones Produced

Melatonin; this hormone is also synthesized in the retina and the gut.

Function of Hormones

Melatonin aids in falling asleep and in getting a deep and refreshing sleep.

Interaction with Other Glands

Through a complex system, light regulates the pineal gland through the retinohypothalamic tract. This tract allows darkness to stimulate production of melatonin and light to inhibit its production.

Taking melatonin as a supplement for sleep is not recommended. First, like all other hormone replacements, by substituting for the function of the gland, the natural production of the gland is decreased by as much as 40%. This is a partial suppression, not total as might happen with high-dose prednisone therapy. Some authors say this suppression is temporary (Hertoghe, 2006). That statement makes no sense to this author. If the hormone replacement therapy continues then the suppressive activity that the hormone exerts on the gland continues. In addition, a high melatonin level can suppress cortisol, suppress the ovaries to the point where it is not recommended for use in pregnancy and can cause hyperthyroidism by facilitating the conversion of T4 to T3.

Signs and Symptoms of Disorder or Dysfunction

Any disturbance involving sleep should raise suspicion of pineal involvement. These symptoms include difficulty falling asleep, difficulty staying asleep, restless legs, tiredness during the day from failure to get restful sleep.

Testing Function

Two tests are available. You can test melatonin directly in the saliva, which allows for serial sampling through the day to track the circadian rhythm. In addition, melatonin and its primary metabolite (6-sulfatoxymelatonin) can be tested in a 24-hour urine sample. This test does show the function of the pineal gland, but because it is all the melatonin and metabolite produced in 24 hours, it loses the ability to track the circadian rhythm.

Therapy

Acupuncture

The main point is GV-20 (*Bai Hui*, Hundred Meetings) at the top of the head if a line were drawn between the tops of the ears.

Secondary points are to calm hyperfunction:

- K-1 (*Yong Quan*, Gushing Spring) on the bottom of the foot.
- To stimulate function K-7 (*Fu Liu*, Returning Current) on the medial ankle.
- Bl-8 (*Lou Que*, Declining Connection) 0.5 cun posterior to GV-20 and 1.5 cun of the midline on both sides.

Homeopathy

The use of homeopathic remedies for the pineal gland is sketchy at best. One of the main remedies is *Ficus religiosa* also called the banyan tree. Buddha sat below this tree when he became enlightened. The fig has a resemblance to the shape of the pineal gland. Also, *Ficus indica*; both these figs are said to contain elements very similar to serotonin.

The use of the French system might be the most efficacious in terms of treating the pineal with homeopathy.

The British pharmacies carry a large selection of potencies of pineal.

Gland Cell Therapy

This is not a popular glandular and may be difficult to find. The suggested amounts for therapy are:

- Oral $\frac{1}{10}$ gm, 3 times a day (Spring, 1921).
- Oral $\frac{1}{10}$ to $\frac{1}{2}$ gm, 3 times day (6 to 30 mg; Harrower, 1922).

Manipulative Therapy

Use spinal-level C1 for chiropractic or osteopathic manipulation and spondylotherapy.

To use Manaka metronome technique, select kidney meridian, 120 beats per minute, on any or all of the above-mentioned acupuncture points.

Color Therapy

Chakra System

Indigo between the eyebrows.

Sound

Chakra system tone B.

Neural Therapy

The main neural point is GV-20 at the crown of the head. Inject 0.50 cc of procaine or if inflammation is suspected also 0.50 cc Traumeel®.

Nutrition

Any food containing tryptophan will help with hormone synthesis. In many treatment strategies, precursors are used such as tryptophan or 5-HTP as individual supplements. These supplements require other components to catalyze the reaction of hormone synthesis or to metabolize the by-products of the reactions. If these products are given alone, the body must provide the other nutrients needed to complete the reaction. This creates a deficiency of the other components of the metabolic process.

A better strategy is to use the most complete nutrient form available so as not to create a deficiency of other nutrients not supplemented. A completely balanced amino acid supplement is best used here. Standard Process Nutrimere® is a good choice because it is a complete protein. Not only does it have precursors to melatonin like tryptophan, it also contains other amino acids to complete the metabolic process. One caution: Nutrimere does come from shellfish.

Light/Dark Cycle Regulation (Additional Therapy)

One very good strategy for balancing the pineal is to completely regulate the light/dark cycles. The first step is to make sure the patient is sleeping in an adequately darkened room. The room should be as dark as possible, even to the point of using black drapes. The pineal patient must never use a night light. This is also a good suggestion for children as a preventative against developing pineal problems.

The second step is to expose the patient to bright light upon arising. The combination of a dark room for sleeping and bright light in the morning will reset the pineal to produce melatonin at night and dramatically slow its production in the morning.

18 Pancreas

Function and Biochemistry

Location: Posterior wall of abdomen.
Size: 12.5 to 15 cm.
Weight: 60 to 100 gm, islet cells 0.9 to 1.5 gm.
Structure: A compound gland, the endocrine function of the outer islet cells is to excrete insulin directly into the bloodstream. The exocrine function is to excrete digestive enzymes into the small intestine.

Hormones Produced

- Alpha cells—glucagons
- Beta cells—insulin
- Delta cells—somatostatin
- Pp cells—pancreatic polypeptide.

Insulin is pulsatile every 1.5 to 2 hours and oscillatory every 6 to 18 minutes; this is one reason diabetes is such a difficult condition to manage with injected insulin. The diabetic is trying to compensate for the lack of this complex and little understood rhythm with a shot of insulin after meals.

Signs and Symptoms of Disorder or Dysfunction

Most people who seek the advice of an integrative endocrinologist will already know their diagnosis if they have Type 1 diabetes. The common symptoms of undiagnosed Type 1 diabetes are easy to recognize. Remember that these signs and symptoms may arise almost overnight. They are increased urination, thirst, hunger, fatigue, irritability, and decreased weight and blurry vision. Immediately test anyone presenting with these symptoms.

Proteins leaking out of the gut (leaky gut syndrome) into the bloodstream are increasingly implicated as a cause of Type 1 diabetes, especially if it is adult onset.

This condition is latent autoimmune diabetes of the adult (LADA). As the proteins leak out of the gut into the bloodstream, they encounter the immune system. At this point, the immune system is very active attacking the dietary proteins. With the immune system in high gear, it is looking for other invading proteins and attacks the pancreas islet cells as a foreign protein. This attack decreases the ability of the islet cells to produce insulin. Recognizing the condition early, a program of oral tolerance is effective. If the autoimmune assault has the opportunity to destroy the islet cells then administering insulin is the only choice. A form of Type 1 diabetes is the result.

Another common problem involving the pancreas is metabolic syndrome. This illness is a high-circulating blood glucose and high insulin level. One common cause is a diet rich in simple carbohydrates beyond the amount needed for life.

The pancreas produces insulin to help metabolize the sugars. As the body develops Type 2 diabetes, the body cells stop recognizing the insulin and the sugars cannot enter the body cells for metabolism.

If not used for body energy these sugars must be stored. They are commonly deposited as abdominal fat, one of the key characteristics of metabolic syndrome.

If there is a problem with the exocrine function of the pancreas, the symptom is indigestion 1 to 2 hours after a meal with nonodorous flatulence.

Testing Function

The first test for diabetes is the fasting plasma glucose test (FPG) commonly called a blood sugar test. This test is done after fasting overnight and the result is the amount of glucose in the blood at the moment of the test. The American Diabetes Association (ADA) states that a test result of 100 to 125 mg/dl is prediabetes. A fasting glucose over 126 mg/dl is a diagnosis of diabetes. The FPG should occur with similar numbers on 2 consecutive days to be a valid diagnosis. The FPG test is included on most regular blood chemistry panels.

Another test for diabetes is the oral glucose tolerance test (OGTT). This test is run after a fast and after drinking a high glucose drink. Blood glucose is measured before the test and 2 hours after the drink. According to the ADA, a blood glucose of 140 to 199 mg/dl is prediabetes and a blood glucose of 200 mg/dl or more is diagnosed as diabetes. This test can also be done at home by simply eating a high carbohydrate meal and checking the blood glucose with a blood glucose meter available at any drug store. For a more accurate picture of the body's reaction to carbohydrates, the testing of the blood glucose can be done every half hour for 5 hours after the meal.

Another common test to determine glucose control is glycosylated hemoglobin (HgbA$_{1c}$). This is a measure of how much glucose is incorporated into the red blood cells. The red blood cells normally live about 120 days; so determining how much glucose is in them gives an idea of what the blood glucose level is on average for 120 days.

Obesity is commonly measured as the body mass index (BMI). This number is determined by a simple calculation that measures weight in proportion to height. Calculate by multiplying weight in pounds by 703, then divide this number by height in inches squared.

$$BMI = Weight\ (lbs) \times 703\ /\ Height^2\ (in)$$

A normal BMI is 18.5 to 24.9; 25 is overweight and obesity begins at 30. Measuring BMI on clients is helpful because it gives them a tangible measure of their situation.

Therapy

Acupuncture

- Bl-13 (*Fei Shu*, Lung Shu) 1.5 cun lateral to lower border of third thoracic vertebra.
- Bl-20 (*Pi Shu*, Spleen Shu) 1.5 cun lateral to the lower border of the eleventh thoracic vertebra.
- Bl-23 (*Shen Shu*, Kidney Shu) 1.5 cun lateral to the lower border of the second lumbar vertebra.
- St-36 (*Zu San Li*, Leg Three Miles) 3 cun inferior to the depressions lateral to the patellar ligament of the knee, 1 cun lateral to the tibia.
- K-3 (*Tai Xi*, Supreme Stream) level with high point of medial malleolus in depression between it and the Achilles tendon.

Auricular Acupuncture

Endocrine and pancreas.

Homeopathy

The *Reference Works®* homeopathic computer program shows 1,282 references and 202 remedies. The main remedies are as follows:

Alloxanum (Allox.). This remedy is a specific for Type 1 diabetes based on its toxicology. It has been used in material doses to induce diabetes experimentally to make it possible to study the disease.

Arsenicum Album (Ars.). The patient who needs *Ars.* is very anxious, even to the point of having panic attacks, especially after midnight. In fact, many of their symptoms are aggravated after midnight. In addition, very fastidious, the patient is chilly and desires heat. Complains of burning pains made better by heat.

Atropine (Atro.). Affinity for the pancreas, hyperesthesia, visual disturbances to the point of illusions, frequent urination, and dry mouth and throat.

Several of the *Calcarea* remedies and several of the *Mercurius* remedies can be indicated.

Iodum (Iod.). Weight loss with great appetite, restlessness, hurried, great weakness, slight exertion brings perspiration, thyroid enlargement.

Iris Versicolor (Iris). Migraine headache, burning the alimentary canal, decreased appetite, nausea, and vomiting.

Natrum Sulphuricum (Nat. Sulph.). Diabetes, especially when combined with asthma. A good remedy for head injury. The author had a case more than 15 years ago where a construction worker was hit in the head with a board while on a job site 20 years earlier and developed headaches and Type 1 diabetes. After one dose of *Nat. Sulph.* 200c and *Nat. Sulph.* 30c once a day for 1 month, he no longer had headaches and no longer needed insulin or any other medicine to control his blood sugar.

Phosphorus (Phos.). Effervescent, excitable, and difficulty with personal boundaries. Examples of the boundary issues are sympathetic leading to empathy severe enough to actually feel the pain or experience the thoughts of others. Very suggestible, with many fears.

Uranium Nitricum (Uran. Nit.). This is another specific for diabetes, creating it in material doses.

Lycopodium (Lyc.) Low self-esteem but with seeming self-confidence, a false bravado. Strong desire for sweets. Many fears. Averse to company but fears being alone. Intellectual with physical weakness.

Syzygium Jambolanum. A specific for diabetes. The dose as listed in Boericke is unusual for a homeopathic remedy. The seeds, powdered, 10 grains (600 mg) 3 times a day or the tincture.

Gland Cell Therapy

Dose:
- Oral, 10 to 30 grains, 3 times a day, 30 minutes to 1 hour after meals; injection, 0.5 to 4 cc once a day (Wolf, 1940).
- Oral, 2 to 8 grains, 3 times a day (Spring, 1921).
- Oral, 5 to 10 grains, 3 times a day (Harrower, 1929).

The Standard Process® line is very helpful when dealing with the pancreas and blood sugar issues.

- Pancreatrophin PMG® 95 mg per tablet of bovine pancreas.
- Paraplex® pancreas, adrenal, pituitary, and thyroid PMG extracts.
- Diaplex® is a combination product of pancreas PMG and cytosol extract plus chromium, betaine hydrochloride, and pancreatin 3x.

Manipulative Therapy

Use spinal-level T6, T7, T8 for chiropractic or osteopathic manipulation and spondylotherapy.

To use Manaka metronome technique, select bladder meridian 112 beats per minute and Stomach 132 beats, on any or all of the above-mentioned acupuncture points.

Nutrition

Diet regulation is extremely important for the person with diabetes. This author advocates a higher protein, lower carbohydrate approach. In the early years of my association with Dr. Steven K. Gordon ND, I watched this approach change the lives of those who suffered with life-long diabetes. He taught each patient the physiology of their disease and, therefore, gave them a reason to comply with dietary guidelines. Testing their blood sugar levels many times a day, they maintain a tight control over those levels with diet regulation and insulin.

The book *Diabetes Solution* by Dr. Richard K. Bernstein MD is a detailed discussion in nonprofessional's language designed to teach diabetic patients everything they need to know to maintain effective blood glucose control. This book is necessary for all practitioners treating diabetics and their patients.

Western Herbal Medicine

- Cinnamon: the journal *Diabetes Care* recommends 1 to 6 gm per day for Type 2 diabetes to reduce blood glucose.
- Juniper berry, uva ursi, shepherd's purse, barberry.

Neural Therapy

Injection into the related spinal levels T6, 7, 8.

Related acupuncture points especially include SP-6.

Color Therapy

Dinshah System

- Lemon systemic front; yellow areas #6, 7, 8, 9, 10, magenta systemic front from #22 (Dinshah, 1980).
- Acute pancreatitis: turquoise systemic front.
- Chronic pancreatitis: lemon systemic front and on #18, yellow on #6–8.
- Hypoglycemia or chronic hyperinsulinemia: lemon systemic.
- Diabetes mellitus Types 1 and 2: lemon systemic front; yellow #6, 7, 8, 9, 10, magenta systemic front from #22.

Chinese Medicinals

- *Yeu Chung* Pills, 6 gm of pills, 4 times a day.
- *Yu Quan Wan*, dose is variable depending on the brand.
- *Xiao Ke Wan*, dose is variable depending on brand.

Sound

The basic sound for the pancreas is D.

If using sound at the same time as the spectrochrome colors: lemon, B; Yellow, A#; Magenta, G and E.

A Case History

This is a very interesting story of a great spokesperson for diabetes.

Eva Saxl a Czechoslovakian Jew who escaped the Nazis in World War II and went to Shang Hai was diagnosed with Type 1 diabetes. In 1941 the Japanese closed the pharmacies in Shang Hai and insulin was only available on the black market. Her husband, Victor, a textile engineer, was able to manufacture insulin from the pancreases of water buffalo and pigs enough to keep his wife Eva and 400 other people in Shang Hai alive for the duration of the war. She went on to become a spokesperson for diabetes until her death in 2004. She was 83 and had diabetes without complications for 60 years.

19 Testes

Function and Biochemistry

Location: In the scrotal sac of the male.
Size: In the adult male, 4.6 cm long, 2.6 cm wide, 18 to 30 cc volume.
Structure: Two cell types, Sertoli cells, and the interstitial Leydig cells.

Hormones Produced

The Sertoli cells produce sperm cells. The Leydig cells produce testosterone, antimullerian hormone, inhibin, activin, and prodynorphin. Also transferrin, which is essential for spermatogenesis.

Function of Hormones

GnRH from the hypothalamus regulates LH and FSH in a pulsatile manner—yet another example of why it is so difficult to recreate bodily hormonal fluctuations with exogenous hormones. When there are pulses of LH and FSH, this creates pulses of testosterone. Administering testosterone as an exogenous hormone, it is given as an injection on an occasional basis, as a transdermal cream administered once a day or as a patch, delivering testosterone at a predetermined continuous rate. "Under ordinary circumstances, LH is exquisitely sensitive to the feedback effects of testosterone, with almost complete suppression after the administration of amounts of exogenous androgen that approximate the normal daily secretory rate of testosterone (~20μmol or 6mg)" (Braunwald *et al.*, 2001).

Interaction with Other Glands

The Leydig cells produce androgenic steroids and are controlled by leutenizing hormone from the pituitary. LH pulses at about the rate of every 1 to 2 hours.

The Sertoli cells produce sperm and are controlled by follicle-stimulating hormone from the pituitary. The secretion of LH and FSH is controlled by the release of gonadotropin-releasing hormone (GnRH) from the hypothalamus.

Signs and Symptoms of Disorder or Dysfunction

There are some testicular dysfunctions that are genetic, like Klinefelter's syndrome. Others involve testosterone resistance, like Reifenstein's syndrome. These diseases are very interesting and can show dramatic symptoms but are beyond the scope of integrative endocrinology. Most cases will center on the problems of aging and the consequences of slowly decreasing testosterone. These include decrease libido, erectile dysfunction, decrease in muscle strength. Another common problem that is not easily dealt with using ordinary medicine is male infertility. The symptoms can be very subtle. The onset of symptoms can take place over many years and may not be recognized until they are dramatic.

Testing Function

Blood tests are available for testosterone, LH, and FSH. Using this combination of tests, diagnosis of testicular disorders is straightforward. Serial saliva sampling is available to track the circadian rhythm of testosterone secretion. Testosterone and its metabolites are tested in the 24-hour urine hormone profile.

Therapy

Acupuncture

- Lv-5 (*Li Gou*, Woodworm Canal) 5 cun above the medial malleolus, just behind the tibia.
- Sp-6 (*San Yin Jiao*, Three Yin Intersection) 3 cun above the medial malleolus just behind the tibia.
- St-44 (*Nei Ting*, Inner Courtyard) between the second and third toe 0.5 cun proximal to the web.

Homeopathy

Agnus Castus (Agn.). The person who needs this remedy is in a very broken-down state with especially low sexual vitality and anxiety about health. Forgetful and absentminded. Impotence.

Lycopodium (Lyc.). Slowly developing conditions with decreased functional power often with liver problems and digestive disturbance, lack of self-confidence, weak memory, impotence, and premature emission.

Phosphoric Acid (Phos. Ac.). Marked debility, use when system is exposed to ravages of acute disease, excesses of activity, alcohol or drugs, grief, and loss of vital fluids.

A traveling sales man came to the clinic with impotence and extreme fatigue. His lifestyle and job did not have any extraordinary features until asked about diet. Drinking two to three six-packs of cola drinks per day while he was driving from customer to customer gave him a tremendous dose of phosphoric acid. Striking the author as very unusual, the *Materia Medica* was consulted. This is an excellent example of the homeopathic principle of material dose of a remedy creating symptoms that are cured by a microdose. Simply stopping his massive intake of phosphoric acid and giving *Phos. Ac.* 30c as a remedy cured the problem.

Gland Cell Therapy

- Oral 2–10 gm, 4 times a day (Spring, 1921).
- Oral 1–10 gm, 3 times a day; injection 1 ampule several times a week (the amount of fresh gland equivalent is variable from 0.5 gm to 15 gm) (Wolf, 1940).
- Oral, 5–15 gm, 3 times a day (Harrower, 1922).
- Injectable 1 cc daily or every other day. Contains 27 gm raw tissue equivalent (Harrower, 1922).

Standard Process® has three products for the male glandular system.

- Symplex M®, this is a male combination glandular; each tablet contains 45 mg bovine orchic PMG, 15 mg bovine adrenal PMG, 10 mg bovine pituitary PMG, and 10 mg bovine thyroid PMG.
- Orchex®, each tablet contains 88 mg bovine orchic cytosol extract.
- Orchic PMG®, each tablet contains 165 mg bovine orchic PMG extract.

Manipulative Therapy

For chiropractic or osteopathic manipulation or spondylotherapy, use L4, L5, and sacrum.

Western Herbal Medicine

- Ginseng (*Panax ginseng*)
- Sarsaparilla (*Smilax officinalis*)
- Saw Palmetto (*Serenoa serrulata*)
- Damiana (*Turnera aphrodisiaca*)
- Yohimbe (*Pausinystalia johimbe*).

Neural Therapy

Injection with a fine needle into the spermatic cord or directly into the testicle. Injection directly into the prostate gland.

Color Therapy

Chakra System

Decreased activity only: red on base chakra areas 10 and 11.

Dinshah System

- Decreased activity: green and orange systemic front, magenta systemic front and on #18, scarlet on # 10 and 11.
- Overactivity: turquoise systemic front, purple on #10, 11, 12, magenta systemic front.

Chinese Medicinals

Many remedies are available for the male glandular system. In Fratkin's book (Fratkin, 2001) alone there are 13 patents made of only plant material and 19 that use plant and animal ingredients.

- Five Ancestors Tea Pills (*Wu Zi Yan Zong Wan*).
- Nine Seeds Returning to Spring Pill (*Jiu Zi Hui Chun Wan*).
- Excessively Limp Effective Remedy (*Kang Wei Ling*).
- Tonify Kidney Pills (*Bou Shen Wan*).
- Man's Treasure (*Xiong Bao*).
- Sea Horse Pills (*Hai Ma Bu Shen Wan*).

Sound

Base chakra sound is C.

20 Ovary

Function and Biochemistry

Aids the growth and development of uterus, vagina, and mammary glands at puberty, secondary sex characteristics, and maintaining the menstrual cycle by the cyclic production of estradiol and progesterone. Production of ova for reproduction.

Location: High on both sides of the female pelvis one ovary on each side, near the posterior wall.
Size: 2 to 5 cm wide, 1.5 to 3 cm long, 0.5 to 1.5 cm thick.
Weight: 10 to 20 gm.
Structure:

- Cortex (contains follicles for ova production)
- Medulla.

Hormones Produced

- Estradiol, the most potent estrogen
- Estrone, some produced in ovary but most is from conversion of androstenedione in peripheral tissues
- Estriol, formed from estrone and estradiol
- Progesterone, secreted by corpus luteum
- Dehydroepiandrosterone (DHEA)
- Androstenadione
- Testosterone
- Dihydrotestosterone
- Inhibin
- Activin
- Follistatin
- Relaxin

Function of Hormones

The estrogens are responsible for secondary sex characteristics in women. They help keep vaginal mucosa thick, thin cervical mucus, and help duct development in the breast.

Progesterone prepares the uterus for implantation of a fertilized egg. Starts the shedding reaction of the uterine lining. It inhibits uterine contraction, thickens cervical mucous, stimulates glandular development in the breast, and increases the body temperature.

Interaction with Other Glands

The hormone products of the ovary act on nearly every tissue in the body. The ovary is controlled by negative feedback with the hypothalamus and pituitary.

Signs and Symptoms of Disorder or Dysfunction

Most patients will come for natural treatment of the female system for one of three reasons. They will come for menopause and its concomitant symptoms, irregular menstruation or infertility. The treatment of all these conditions is similar. Integrative endocrinology only seeks to balance the system. We are not manipulating function by administering hormones or drugs. Each of these conditions involves the interplay of incredibly complex hormonal interactions. In integrative endocrinology, we seek to harmonize this glandular communication. The female endocrine disorders are some of the most fascinating because these conditions give us opportunities when we can truly witness the healing power of nature. By using very simple and broad therapeutic application, we witness dramatic changes in health.

The symptomatic definition of menopause is no menstrual period for 1 year. Confirm menopause by serum evaluation of FSH, LH, and estradiol. The FSH and LH should be elevated and the estradiol decreased.

Laboratory evaluation will sometimes show the hormone imbalance causing heavy, irregular, or painful menses. Often, the symptoms will be your only guide.

In infertility, medical evaluation is necessary because often there is a mechanical problem like a blocked fallopian tube. Ruling out mechanical difficulties or dramatic hormone imbalances, there is much to be gained by a functional integrative approach.

Medically evaluating heavy or painful menses is important because there may be a pathological underlying cause. A gynecologic exam and laboratory evaluation are essential.

Therapy

Acupuncture

- Sp-6 (*San Yin Jiao*, Three Yin Intersection) 3 cun above the medial malleolus just behind the tibia.
- St-44 (*Nei Ting*, Inner Courtyard) between the second and third toe 0.5 cun proximal to the web.
- LI-4 (*He Gu*, Joining Valley) hold the thumb and forefinger together; the point is at the highest point of the first interosseous muscle.
- Bl-32 (*Ci Liao*, Second Crevice).

Homeopathy

If you are not a trained homeopath, the author recommends using the French method or making a referral. A check of the words ovary, menses, menopause, and infertility in the *Reference Works*® homeopathic computer program yields 2,438 remedies and 98,185 references.

Gland Cell Therapy

- Oral ovary 5 to 10 gm twice a day, fresh organ may be used 10 to 15 gm (Sajous, 1992).
- Oral 2 to 20 gm, 3 times a day; injection 1 cc equals 1 to 22 gm of tissue (Wolf, 1940).
- Oral 2 to 4 gm, 3 times a day (Spring, 1921).
- Oral 2 to 5 gm, 3 times a day (Harrower, 1922).

Standard Process® products:

- Symplex F® is a female combination glandular; each tablet contains 30 mg bovine ovary PMG, 15 mg bovine adrenal PMG, 10 mg bovine pituitary PMG®, and 10 mg bovine thyroid PMG. The usual starting dose is 1 tablet, 3 times a day. This dose is low compared to historical doses.
- Ovex®, each tablet contains 120 mg of bovine ovary cytosol extract.
- Ovex p®, each tablet contains 120 mg of porcine ovary cytosol extract.
- Ovatrophin PMG®, each tablet contains 125 mg of bovine ovary PMG extract.

Manipulative Therapy

Use L4, L5, and sacrum for chiropractic or osteopathic manipulation and spondylotherapy.

Western Herbal Medicine

Menopausal symptoms:

- Black cohosh (*Cimicifuga racemosa*)
- Chaste tree (*Vitex agnus-castus*)
- Kava (*Piper methysticum*).

Menstrual disorders added to the above herbs:

- Ginger (*Zingiber officinal*).

Neural Therapy

If presented with abdominal symptoms of gynecologic origin, it is useful to palpate the abdominal musculature for sensitive areas. Often, complaints that appear to arise from inside the abdomen are actually from the hyperalgetic abdominal wall. This painful spot on the abdominal wall may be the origin of the problem or, as was discussed in the acupuncture chapter, there is a two-way communication between the internal organs and the body surface by way of the acupuncture meridian system. In addition to the regular meridians, there are a number of recognized pathways in the acupuncture system as shown on acupuncture charts. These include the internal pathway of the main meridian, the lou connecting channel, the divergent channel, and the sinew channel. Each of these channels exists for each of the 12 organ meridians. These are established pathways of energy movement. Therefore, the sensation of an internal disorder is easily transmitted to the surface of the body and the energy of a therapeutic intervention at the surface of the body is easily transmitted to the interior.

Color Therapy

Chakra System

Decreased activity: only red on base chakra areas 10 and 11.

Dinshah System

- Menopausal complaints: green and magenta, systemic front and #18.
- Decreased activity: green and orange systemic front, magenta systemic front and on #18, scarlet on #10 and 11.
- Overactivity: turquoise systemic front: purple on #10, 11, 12, magenta systemic front.

Chinese Medicinals

- *Dong Quai* (*Angelica sinensis*). This herb is a great female tonic.

Menopausal formulas:

- Restorative Pills (*He Che Da Zao Wan*).
- Two Immortals Tea Pills (*Er Xian Tan Wan*).

Difficult menses with cold signs:

- Crampbark Plus (*Tong Jing Wan*) from Health Concerns®.

Difficult menses with heat signs:

- Unlocking from Health Concerns®.

Excessive menstrual bleeding:

- With cold signs: Longevitabs and Postpartum from Health Concerns®.
- With heat signs: Unlocking and Formula H from Health Concerns®.

Infertility:

- With cold signs: Maternal Herbal from Health Concerns®.
- Yin deficiency: Fertile Garden from Health Concerns®.

Sound

Base chakra sound is C.

21 Thymus Gland

Function and Biochemistry

The thymus gland is responsible for the production of T lymphocytes that are one of the main components of the immune system.

Location: In the chest, behind the sternum.
Size: Length 5 cm, width 4 cm, thickness 6 cm, these are the dimensions at birth.
Weight: At birth 15 gm increasing to 35 gm at puberty and then going through an involution process at 60 years, 15 gm and at 70 years, 0 gm.
Structure: A medulla of epithelial cells and a cortex of lymphoid cells.

Hormones Produced

Thymopoietin and thymosin; these are growth factors to direct the maturation of T cells.

Function of Hormones

The main hormones are responsible for the development of T lymphocytes. Immature thymocites progress through the gland from the cortex to the medulla, maturing along the way. These lymphocytes are then released into the circulation.

Interaction with Other Glands

The involution process is said to be governed by increasing circulation of sex hormones; however, the involution process does not seem to reverse with aging and declining sex hormones.

Signs and Symptoms of Disorder or Dysfunction

A decrease in immune function can be a sign of underactivity of the thymus. An autoimmune disorder can signal the need to regulate the thymus.

Testing Function

The laboratory evaluation of the thymus gland involves a level of immunological testing that goes beyond the scope of this text. Treatment of the thymus can proceed in integrative endocrinology without this complex level of testing because our methods are not dependent on the exact criteria required for evaluation of the function of the gland but can function on the fact of an immunological insult to the body. These problems can be infection from an external pathogen or an autoimmune assault. These circumstances demand an intervention with appropriate measures from an integrative endocrinology standpoint.

Therapy

Acupuncture

- ST-11 (*Qi She*, Abode of Qi) in the depression between the sternal head and the clavicular head of the sternocleidomastoid muscle.
- P-6 (*Nei Guan*, Inner Pass) on ventral part of the wrist 2 cun proximal to the wrist crease between the tendon palmaris longus and flexor carpi radialis.

Both the above points can be used for any thymus problems using either a tonifying or a sedating manipulation of the point.

- HT-9 (*Shao Chong*, Lesser Rushing) at the ungueal angle of the little finger, medial side. Tonification point.
- HT-7 (*Shen Men*, Spirit Gate) at the wrist crease on the radial side of the flexor carpi ulnaris tendon, sedation point.

Homeopathy

Reference Works® shows 274 references and 44 remedies. Most of the references are not extensive except for the use of homeopathic thymus, used according to the French system.

Viscum Album (mistletoe). This remedy might be difficult to prescribe for the thymus because of the paucity of symptoms. Symptoms include difficulty breathing, worse lying on the left side. Weight and oppression around the heart.

Gland Cell Therapy

Standard Process® products:

- Thymex® is a whole gland product containing 130 mg of cytosol extract.
- Thymus PMG® is the protomorphogen that is a thymus builder 185mg.
- Congaplex® contains 120 mg thymus cytosol extract. This product is excellent for any infection from any source.

Western Herbal Medicine

- *Echinacea angustifolia*, 1 to 3 gm/day dried root; 2 to 6 ml/day, 1:2 liquid extract.
- *E. purpurea*, 2.5 to 6 gm/day dried aerial parts.

Neural Therapy

Use related acupuncture points and CV-17 in the middle of the sternum at the fourth intercostals space.

Color Therapy

Chakra System

Heart chakra: green color.

Dinshah System

- Thymus atrophy: lemon systemic front.
- Thymus hypertrophy: lemon systemic front, indigo on 4 to 5.

Sound

Tone F.

Manipulative Therapy

Use spinal-level C7, T1, T2, T3 for chiropractic or osteopathic manipulation and spondylotherapy.

   To use Manaka metronome technique, select pericardium meridian, 176 beats per minute and heart meridian 126 beats on any or all of the above-mentioned acupuncture points. In addition, use sternal tapping with the Manaka heart frequency.

22 Parathyroid Gland

Function and Biochemistry

The parathyroid glands are responsible for regulating calcium metabolism.

Location: Posterior surface of lobes of the thyroid gland in the neck.
Size: 6 to 8 mm long and 3 to 4 mm wide, 4 separate glands.
Weight: Variable; based on blood calcium level, the number of cells can dramatically increase with low calcium, low vitamin D ($1,25(OH)_2 D_3$), or high phosphates.
Structure: Granular epithelial cells with vascular connective tissue.

Hormones Produced

Parathyroid hormone (PTH). The glands can rapidly secrete stored hormone, synthesize and store large amounts of hormone, or they can increase in size if there is low calcium or vitamin D3 in the blood stream. This allows the parathyroid glands to respond to any situation of calcium increase or decrease in the blood stream whether chronic or acute.

Function of Hormones

Binds to receptors in the surface of bone and kidney cells increasing blood calcium. PTH also increases kidney synthesis of vitamin D3.

Interaction with Other Glands

Calcium and vitamin D3 in the blood signal the parathyroid to decrease production of PTH. The parathyroid glands interact with the bones, kidneys, and intestines.

Signs and Symptoms of Disorder or Dysfunction

Hyperfunction is characterized by hypercalcemia; hypophosphatemia increases urinary output of calcium; and phosphate increases alkaline phosphatase, hyposensitivity in the neuromuscular system, and demineralization of the skeleton. Recurrent kidney stones may also be a sign of parathyroid problems.

Testing function: Serum level of PTH can be tested.

Therapy

Acupuncture

- ST-9 (*Ren Ying*, Man's Welcome) 1.5 cun lateral to the tip of the laryngeal prominence. Caution: The carotid artery underlies this point.

For Hypoparathyroidism Add

- TW-3 (*Zhong Zhu*, Central Islet) dorsum of the hand between the fourth and fifth metacarpal bones just proximal to the metacarpalphalageal joint.
- LI-4 (*He Gu*, Joining Valley) hold the thumb and forefinger together; the point is at the highest point of the first interosseous muscle.

For Hyperparathyroidism Add

- ST-44 (*Nei Ting*, Inner Courtyard) just proximal to the web margin between the second and third toe.
- LV-3 (*Tai Chong*, Great Rushing) top of the foot in the hollow distal to the junction of the first and second metatarsal bones. Usually the dorsalis pedis artery can be felt pulsing.

Homeopathy

Reference Works® shows 77 references and 18 remedies. These references are to the parathyroid used as in the French method and some of the calcium-based remedies.

Gland Cell Therapy

- Oral, 0.5 gm, 5 to 8 per day (Sajous, 1992). Sajous also mentions the method of Berkeley where he obtains the glands fresh at the abattoirs under his supervision. The glands are minced and 5 to 8 glands are given in a bread and butter sandwich once a day.
- Oral, 1/10 to 0.5 gm, 3 times a day; injectable, 50 to 1000 IU once a day. Blood calcium must be checked to avoid overdose (Wolf, 1940).
- Oral 1/20 to 1/10 gm, 2 to 3 times a day (Spring, 1921).
- Standard Process® Cal-ma Plus®, 3 tablets supply 2.3 mg parathyroid.

Manipulative Therapy

Use spinal-level C6 and C7 for chiropractic or osteopathic manipulation.
For spondylotherapy use spinal-level C6 and C7.

To use Manaka metronome technique, select triple-burner meridian, 152 beats per minute and stomach 132 beats, on any or all of the above-mentioned acupuncture points.

Color Therapy

Chakra System

Blue on throat area.

Dinshah System

- Hypoparathyroid: lemon systemic front, indigo on #3.
- Hyerparathyroidism: lemon and orange systemic front.

Sound

Tone G.

23 Liver

Function and Biochemistry

The liver performs many functions, including synthesis of albumin, proteins, coagulation factors, hormonal and growth factors, bile acids, cholesterol, lecithin, phospholipids. It also regulates glucose, glycogen, lipids, cholesterol, and amino acids. The liver is responsible for filtration and elimination of many toxins and drugs.

Location: Right upper quadrant of the abdomen.
Size: Largest organ in the body, not including the skin.
Weight: 1 to 1.5 kg.
Structure: Two-thirds of the liver is hepatocytes. The remaining cells are the reticuloendothelial Kupffer cells, stellate and endothelial cells, blood vessels, and bile duct cells.

Hormones Produced

*   Insulin-like growth factor 1 (IGF-1) (somatomedin)
*   Angiotensinogen
*   Thrombopoietin (TPO).

The liver clears, regulates, metabolizes, and converts many of the body hormones.

Function of Hormones

IGF-1 stimulates body growth. Angiotensinogen is a precursor to angiotensin, which controls blood pressure.

Thrombopoieten helps generate platelets.

Interaction with Other Glands

Pituitary growth hormone binds to receptors on liver cells stimulating the release of IGF-1. Insulin from the pancreas causes the liver to store glucose as glycogen.

Signs and Symptoms of Disorder or Dysfunction

Bedside diagnostic signs are pain in liver region, jaundice, and difficulty digesting fat. If there is a developed liver problem usually fat intake will cause diarrhea.

Liver enzyme tests are an inexpensive liver diagnostic tool; they are as follows:

- Aspartate aminotransferase (AST) increase can occur if other tissues in addition to the liver are injured.
- Alanine aminotransferase (ALT) is specific to the liver.
- Gamma-glutamyltransferase (GGT) helps to monitor biliary obstruction.
- Alkaline phosphatase to monitor bile duct obstruction.

These liver enzymes are released into the blood when liver cells are injured or destroyed.

Therapy

Acupuncture

- St-36 (*Zu San Li*, Leg Three Miles) 3 cun inferior to the depressions lateral to the patellar ligament of the knee, 1 cun lateral to the tibia. Liver support.
- Sp-6 (*San Yin Jiao*, Three Yin Intersection) 3 cun above the medial malleolus just behind the tibia. Liver support.
- Lv-2 (*Xing Jian*, Moving Between) dorsum of the foot, between first and second toes, 0.5 cun proximal to the web. Sedates the liver.
- Lv-8 (*Qu Quan*, Spring at the Crook) superior to the medial end of the popliteal crease, in the depression anterior to the tendons of *m. semitendinosus* and *m. semimembranosus*. Tonifies the liver.

Homeopathy

A search of *Reference Works*® yields 26,670 references and 1,145 remedies—obviously a monumental sorting and selection task. The five main remedies are as follows:

Aconitum Napellus (Acon.). To use *Acon*. the symptoms need to include fear and anxiety, including fear of death. It is a strong remedy with a dramatic presentation. The liver symptoms are hot, tense abdomen. Pain not relieved by any position. The author has used this remedy successfully many times for jaundice in newborns.

Lycopodium Clavatum (Lyc.). Right-sided complaints, intellectually strong but physically weak, dictatorial, desire for sweets, easy satiety, pain in abdomen shoots right to left.

Nux Vomica (Nux V.). Nervous, intellectual, overworked, fastidious. Uses a lot of coffee, alcohol, and tobacco. Irritable, portal congestion averse to noise, light, and odor. Has constipation.

Phosphorus (Phos.). Patient is usually tall and slender. Very sensitive to light, sound, even the thoughts of others. Sharp abdominal pain, acute hepatitis, jaundice, and liver congestion.

Sulphur (Sulph.). Irritable, forgetful, selfish, depressed. Hot burning pain, worse from heat and better cold, averse to bathing. Abdomen raw and sore inside, movements as if something alive. Worse in bed at night.

Gland Cell Therapy

- Oral dose equivalent to 10 to 50 gm, 2 to 3 times a day (this means 1 to 5 tablets) injectable, 1 to 3 cc of injection was equal to 10 gm but was only given 1 to 3 times per week (Wolf, 1940).
- Oral, 2 to 5 gm per day (Spring, 1921).
- Oral liver substance, 5 to 10 gm, 3 times a day; anabolin (liver fat extract; Harrower, 1922).
- Standard Process® Livaplex® a combination liver product.
- Hepatrophin PMG® 320 mg per tablet of liver nucleoproteins.
- Dr. Ron's ultra pure freeze-dried liver 500 mg capsules.

Manipulative Therapy

Enervated by the vagus nerve manipulation of C1 and T4 and T9–11.
   Manaka liver 108 beats per minute

Western Herbal Medicine

- *Silybum marianum*
- *Taraxacum officinal radix*
- *Schisandra chinensis.*

Neural Therapy

Inject under the skin to raise a weal at the costal margin over the liver at any area of tenderness and paravertebral points at T9–11.

Color Therapy

Chakra system

Yellow.

Dinshah System

- Acute hepatitis: green and blue systemic front, red on #7 and 8.
- Chronic hepatitis: lemon systemic front, red on 7 and 8, magenta 4, 5, 6, 7, 8, 18, indigo on affected areas if ascites or hemorrhages occur.

Chinese Medicinals

- Minor Bupleurem Decoction Pills (*Xiao Chai Hu Tang Wan*). Cleanses and cools the liver. Symptoms are distention, lymphatic congestion, nausea, hepatitis, and jaundice. Not to be used with hypertension or headaches.
- Bupleurum Dredge Liver Pills (*Chai Hu Shu Gan Wan*). Stagnation of liver qi, abdominal fullness, cold hands and feet, poor circulation, nausea.

24 Hormone Replacement Therapy and Hormone Resistance

Hormone replacement has become the main tool in the practice of medical endocrinology along with a few surgeries and some suppressive and destructive drug therapies.

The *Women's Health Initiative* study set out to determine the safety and efficacy of this type of therapy using synthetic female hormones for menopausal women. The results were a disaster (Chen *et al.*, 2002).

Researchers stopped the study years early because the long-term side effects were much more devastating than the symptoms that synthetic hormone replacement therapy was trying to treat and the long-presumed benefits in the theoretical therapeutic benefits were nowhere to be seen. Because this was the first comprehensive and large-scale study of female hormone replacement therapy (HRT), there were much data gleaned from the study that was previously unknown.

Ordinary medicine had been using these hormones to treat menopausal women for years without actually knowing the side effects. The assumption was that replacing the hormones that were beginning to diminish at menopause would change the signs and symptoms that seemed to be connected to this loss of hormones. Some of these symptoms are hot flashes and night sweats, cardiac problems, and bone loss. The addition of congeated estrogens (the synthetic kind made from pregnant horse urine) helped tremendously with hot flushes and night sweats in most women. However, with estrogen replacement, there were more cardiac events and strokes. Bone loss continued with estrogen administration, and most important, the rate of breast cancer increased tremendously by a factor of 65% to 80% if all histologic types of breast cancer are considered together (Chen *et al.*, 2002).

These dangerous side effects were a surprise to those running the study and to the physicians who were prescribing these synthetic hormones every day. The assumption was that by replacing the missing hormones, the body would automatically stop the processes of aging. Once studied, it turned out to be a false assumption.

Another method of replacing diminishing hormone production is by administering so-called bioidentical hormones. The manufacture of bioidentical hormones is from plant (botanical) sources in the laboratory. Even though they are a pharmaceutical product, their molecular structure is the same as the hormones the body produces. The claim is that these hormones mimic the body's of naturally produced hormones. The replacement of these hormones is supposed to slow down or reverse the symptoms of menopause in women and slow the aging process in men and women.

Research shows that the synthetic replacement of female hormones is devastating to the human body. Is it reasonable to assume that the administration of hormones that are identical to the hormones produced by the body will be safe and effective? To date, no long-term studies have shown this to be true. The assumption of safety and efficacy seems to make sense, but we are still interfering with natural body processes.

Suzanne Somers, a 60-something actor and entrepreneur, is promoting the use of bioidentical hormone replacement through television appearances and popular press books, but studies are not forthcoming to prove the claims made that, since they are identical to what the body produces, they are perfectly safe and effective.

A part of the normal aging process is a slow diminution of hormones over time. As the blood and nerve supply begins to age, the endocrine glands age also. This aging causes a decrease in hormone production. Is it reasonable to take exogenous hormones to reproduce the levels of youth? What will happen to an aging body suddenly catapulted back to age 30 by the stimulation of increasing hormone levels when taking hormones as drugs? Is this like putting jet fuel into a 1947 Chevy? Of course, theoretically it goes like crazy for a while, but what overworked structures are first to break?

The point may not be just the safety of the hormones, but the safety of using anything to bring the body, by chemical force, back to youth. This medical intervention is not gentle rebuilding of structures that, over time, have begun to function less efficiently because of age. Hormone replacement is an instant change, replacing the function of one or usually several endocrine glands back to the levels of their production at approximately age 30 years. This can put stress on nonendocrine tissues that are not used to this high hormone content. The dramatic increase in hormones forces the body's tissues to begin to function at a youthful level, but it also diminishes the function of the gland that produces the hormone. The body interprets the increase in circulating hormone level as indicating that the body is producing enough of the hormone and the gland can work less. This creates a situation of atrophy of the gland.

The fact that HRT is always suppressive to the gland is one of several problems to be addressed before hormone replacement (HRT) is considered. These are serious and undeniable changes to the body with dramatic and lasting effects.

We can use standard thyroid hormone as an example with a well-known and predictable outcome for hormone replacement therapy. First, thyroid-stimulating hormone (TSH), T3, and T4 are tested. T3 and T4 are both available as separate hormones for prescription. Most medical doctors use only levothyroxin, that is, a synthetically produced, bioidentical T4. The hormone is given at a dose level where TSH is suppressed into the normal range and T4 is in the upper half of the normal range. This produces a 30 percent to 40 percent suppression of the thyroid's production of T3 and T4. The reason for this should be obvious: the patient came in with low thyroid hormone output, and the function of the gland has been replaced so the gland is functioning less than it did when first tested. The reason the gland is functioning less is the pituitary secretion of TSH is purposefully suppressed by the administration of T4. Therefore, the thyroid gland is receiving less stimulation from the pituitary. Ordinary medicine realizes that in this situation the patient will have to continue thyroid therapy for life. The only way to remove the thyroid replacement therapy is by an aggressive feeding program that brings the thyroid gradually back to health, while slowly reducing the thyroid replacement. This kind of program slowly increases the ability of the thyroid to produce hormones and allows the pituitary to slowly adjust so that it will not overproduce TSH.

Thyroid hormone replacement therapy is a clear example of bioidentical hormone replacement, giving only physiologic doses to bring the circulating hormone level back to normal. This is the same method used for all bioidentical hormone replacement.

This same glandular involution process occurs with the administration of cortisol, DHEA, prednisone, or dexamethazone. Administering synthetic adrenal cortical hormones (for example, prednisone), is so compromising to the gland that the patient must be followed for a full year after therapy is discontinued. If the patient experiences stress of an emotional nature or severe physical illness, an auto accident, or surgery, they may need to go back on the drug to avoid complete adrenal collapse. The adrenal gland in this situation is so involuted that it probably will not respond to the crisis.

In practice, taking someone off these hormones can be miserable for the patient and the practitioner. First, the patient tests low for one or more hormones. Next, he or she is prescribed a sufficient amount of hormone to replace what was seen on this single test to be lower than the normal range for a 30-year-old. If at this point the patient feels fine, then all is well and he or she can continue with hormone prescribed. If, on the other hand, the patient does not do well on the HRT and attempts to discontinue the prescription on their own, the trouble begins.

The glands related to the prescribed hormones have been suppressed according to the amount of hormone given. If the patient goes off the hormones quickly, they are thrust into a situation worse than the original. This scenario creates a withdrawal situation that must be carefully managed.

Another serious problem with HRT is it is difficult to truly assess the function of the endocrine glands based on any available test. The 24-hour urine hormone profile gives the amounts present in one day's urine sample. The test examines the male and female sex hormones, adrenal hormones, and some of their metabolites. Several assumptions are necessary to rely on this test for hormone replacement therapy. An assumption is made that the patient is functioning normally in regards to the rhythmic nature of their production of hormones. Consider the amount of cortisol produced in one 24-hour period as shown by the test. Is this the amount the patient usually produces on a normal day? If so, it might be fine to give cortisol replacement based on these numbers. If on the other hand this day was abnormal, if the patient had more or less stress, pain, bad news, then the numbers will be skewed and the hormone dose may be grossly incorrect until the next test, which in most clinics is carried out after a year or more. Also, no account is given of the circadian rhythm of cortisol by a 24-hour test, so the clinician must guess when the doses should be administered.

If a serum test is used, then we lose the benefit of knowing the overall production of one day but we do know the precise amount produced at a particular time of day. This means that we must assume as discussed earlier that the patient is producing hormones according to the normal circadian rhythm.

A serial saliva cortisol level may be one answer to these problems. It shows the circadian rhythm of production as well as the total bioavailable hormone produced in one day. However, there is controversy as to the efficacy and accuracy of the test.

Lack of legal regulation is another of the major problems with hormone replacement. Many of these hormones may be purchased over the counter in health food stores in the United States.

Two hormones in this category are dehydroepiandrosterone (DHEA) and melatonin. So much misinformation exists about these hormones and their use that even consumers who think they are informed may be causing themselves a lot of hidden trouble. In the book *DHEA: A Practical Guide*, Dr. Ray Sahelian states (Sahelian, 1996: 9) that there is no feedback mechanism as with other hormones, so taking DHEA will not suppress the body's own production. Later in the same book (p. 110), Sahelian states that DHEA is produced in the zona reticularis of the adrenal gland and is stimulated by ACTH. This kind of confusing information is what the public is getting about HRT.

The body produces around 4 mg per day of DHEA and 7 to 15 mg per day of DHEAS (Williams, 2003). Common supplement doses found in the health food store are 5 mg, 10 mg, 25 mg, and 50 mg. ACTH does stimulate androgen secretion (Williams, 2003). There may also be an additional androgen

(DHEA) stimulating hormone because there can be some differences between the secretory rhythms of cortisol and DHEA, but they show a similar, although not exact, circadian rhythm.

A 50 mg dose of DHEA is more than 12 times the body's normal production. Many doctors are recommending 100 to 150 mg per day, obviously far exceeding the body's natural production of the hormone. If a patient is taking 20 mg, he or she is exceeding the maximum recognized production of the adrenal gland for DHEA and DHEAS. This must have a suppressive action on the pituitary production of ACTH and must, therefore, reduce the production of DHEA and cortisol by the adrenal glands.

Melatonin is not without its problems as it also suppresses cortisol production by the adrenal glands.

There are many questions in ordinary medicine about giving hormones other than those used for menopausal women, such as human growth hormone (HGH).

HGH is a recombinant DNA hormone. Genetic engineering alters a microorganism to produce bioidentical human growth hormone as a by-product of its metabolism. The question arises then, if you are stimulating growth with the addition of exogenous growth hormone, which increases muscle mass and decreases fat among other things, does it stimulate the growth of unwanted tissues like cancer? Because of this concern, and others, ordinary medicine uses human growth hormone only in cases of diagnosed idiopathic short stature and not as a health builder or for antiaging.

Hormone Resistance

Another problem is that the administration of hormones changes the sensitivity of hormone receptors. As the receptors become accustomed to high circulating levels of hormone they are less affected by the hormone. These resistance states can also occur without the administration of exogenous hormones.

There are many recognized states of hormone resistance. The main characteristics of such states are an adequate or even excess compliment of hormone in the blood circulation with symptoms of a hormone deficiency. There is general recognition of some of these states like insulin resistance, which is one component of insulin resistance syndrome also known as metabolic syndrome or syndrome X. In insulin resistance, blood levels of insulin are increased because of dietary intake of sugars leading to a lack of reaction of body cells to insulin. This creates a situation where glucose from the bloodstream cannot enter the cell and so deposits as abdominal fat, among other effects.

There are also some less well-known conditions like thyroid hormone resistance. Resistance to thyroid hormone (RTH), although not often seen, is well documented: "Mutations in the ligand-binging domain of one of the thyroid receptor isoforms (TRb) account for almost all cases" (Yen, 2002).

Another type of hormone resistance comes from the administration of drugs that block the body's absorption of specific hormones like selective serotonin reuptake inhibitors (SSRI) that have the net effect of increasing blood levels of serotonin. There is an escalating medical use of these drugs. The constant exposure of the serotonin receptors to increased levels of serotonin creates a hormone pressure on the receptors. This pressure can lead to a breakdown of the receptors' ability to respond to the hormone. This causes the need to increase the drug dose to continue the desired effect and the potential for a withdrawal syndrome from discontinuing the drug. You can predict how well a person with depression will respond to these drugs by knowing how many times they have used them in the past. The more times these drugs are given, the less effective they are. After a period of time, this situation would make it very difficult to stop taking these drugs because of the precipitous drop in serotonin in the patient's blood stream when the body started to again absorb serotonin normally. In addition, the glandular mechanism for creating serotonin would be suppressed by the high blood levels, and it would have to be stimulated to return to normal after a period of involution.

25 Oral Tolerance/Protomorphology

The premise of oral tolerance (OT) is that an isolated tissue substance, which is taken from an animal and manufactured into a tablet and administered orally, is absorbed and attacked by the immune system. This process only happens if there are already immune cells targeted to that specific tissue. This process diverts the immune cells that are causing a reaction in the body from the original site of the attack to the site of absorption of the oral material. This is true for a food allergen, inhaled pollen, or an autoimmune reaction against the body's own tissues. This process, first described over 100 years ago in 1909 (Besredka, 1909) was further discussed in a 1911 article (Wells and Osborne, 1911).

OT is similar in nature to the idea of protomorphology (PM) proposed by Dr. Royal Lee in 1947. Lee completely outlines his theory in a text of the same name (Lee, 1947). The vital difference in the methods of OT and PM goes to the heart of the reason PM has had better success than OT especially in cases of autoimmune disease.

OT as practiced today uses whole cells. This means, for example, treating a patient with multiple sclerosis by oral administration of pills made of whole nerve cells of bovine or ovine origin.

Lee discovered what he believed to be the organizing principle of cellular structure that he called the protomorphogen (PMG). This organizing principle is a mineral template used to create a cell. To use this PMG for treatment, Lee extracted the PMG from the whole cell by mixing the cells in a hypertonic saline solution. This solution causes the cell wall to break, releasing the nucleus into the solution. Collecting the nuclear material, it is made into a pill. This method seems to be more effective for autoimmune conditions than the administration of whole cell products. The reason PM is superior to OT is probably that the building block of the cell, that is, the protomorphogen, is presented directly to the immune cells, not the surface of the whole cell.

Lee's book was reviewed in the *Journal of the American Medical Association* (Fishbein, 1948). The reviewer wrote that following the author's further discussion and elaboration would not serve a useful purpose. He also wrote that Lee and his coauthor had read widely but not critically and had forced the cited works to fit their theory. In addition, the idea of the body attacking itself had no merit.

Little did the reviewer know that some years later, autoimmunity would be known to be responsible for many diseases and the treatment by animal cells would be at the forefront of research.

The New York Academy of Sciences has issued two books on studies of oral tolerance. Very promising research fills these texts. However, this author must agree with Mark Anderson, a representative of a standard process company for 35 years, who, for at least a decade, has said the failure of OT is not in the practice itself but stems from not feeding the target tissue.

This means that treating a case of Hashimoto's thyroiditis using thyroid gland cell material is not enough. This will temporarily stop the immune attack, thus creating a window of opportunity for healing. Then the practitioner can encourage healing by using the other methods outlined in this book.

The purpose of OT is to stop the autoimmune attack by ingesting the gland cell material and therefore putting that material in contact with the gut-associated lymphoid tissue (GALT).

Using OT in this way is only half the process. Organ-specific nutrition and other healing modalities encourage the rebuilding of the target organ. With the end of tissue destruction, comes the end of stimulation of the immune system.

As practitioners, we may never know why a certain autoimmune process started, but by using the complete method of oral tolerance and gland feeding, whether by specific nutrition or energetic methods like acupuncture to promote healing, these immune attacks against the self may be stopped permanently.

These methods did not originate with Royal Lee. However, Lee codified the practice, introducing a concept of autoimmunity that was previously unknown.

Dr. Harrower's treatment of nausea and vomiting during pregnancy is an interesting example, which goes to show that this method had been used by Harrower before Dr. Lee did. Harrower states that hyperemesis gravidarum is a toxemia in which the placenta puts proteins into the blood stream to which the body reacts unfavorably. The reason for the reaction is the placenta contains genetic material from the mother and father. Perceiving the father's genetic material as foreign, the body mounts an immune attack. Feeding these patients placental substance, a great number improve regardless of the severity of the problem (Harrower, 1922).

The American pharmaceutical manufacturers used to supply this product along with all other gland medicines in the days of Harrower and Wolf. The Chinese pharmacies used to import this product into the United States as recently as 2004. Now the FDA has deemed it unsafe. As an integrative endocrinologist, this does not need to stop you from using these powerful medicines. Many women save the placenta from a previous pregnancy. Dry the placenta in a food dehydrator and encapsulate it. Rarely saved at slaughter, placenta and all other glands are available by contacting an organic farmer. A method that is better than a food dehydrator is a vacuum desiccator. These are available from chemical supply houses at very reasonable prices. Add a small vacuum pump, and you can produce your own glandular remedies for oral tolerance, though medicines produced this way could not be offered for sale; however, even the patient him or herself could be guided to use this method.

Experimentation continues into the mechanisms of oral tolerance. Researchers studying a number of disease states are finding favorable results in many cases. If the practitioner wishes success in the clinic, this author believes that feeding the affected tissue must accompany oral tolerization. OT is one theory that describes how these tissue remedies act in the body. Other theories are presented elsewhere in this text. No matter which theory is the ultimate explanation of action, following the protocols in this book will yield impressive results, as seen for thousands of years, on untold number of patients.

Conclusion

The endocrine glands discussed in this text are the basic structures comprising only a portion of the entire endocrine system. If we concentrate our healing effort on these structures, we have the opportunity to heal the entire system because of the great impact of these structures on all parts of the body and their interaction with the entire endocrine system.

Dr. John Lee liked to say that a fat woman after menopause had just as much estrogen as a skinny woman before menopause. Such is the estrogenic ability of adipose tissue. Fat tissue is now considered by some to be a fully functioning endocrine structure.

Many tissues besides the known and named endocrine glands have an action at a distance by way of hormones. These structures interact with and affect every body tissue. Medically influencing this intricate system is about balance and harmonization, not control. At this time, we do not understand all the endocrine interactions taking place at every second of every day. Nor can we calculate the impact of the use of hormones manufactured in a laboratory on the overall function of the system.

We must rely on the healing power of nature. This statement implies giving the body the minimum of assistance to heal, and to decrease dependence on substances from the outside except food. It also favors removing obstacles to healing.

The more research into endocrine function, the more the number of hormones are discovered in the process, and the more their interaction is uncovered. To think that we as clinicians can really know and appropriately imitate the function of the endocrine system seems unlikely. Hormone production of each gland is rhythmic and pulsitile, often based on unknown factors. This makes substituting the function of a gland by using an exogenous hormone difficult at best. This author believes it is better to help the endocrine system function in a healthy manner, by encouraging optimum glandular activity and without the use of exogenous hormones. Hormones are available as a last resort when an endocrine organ fails. We know that, even at low physiologic replacement doses, we are still suppressing the normal function of the gland and perhaps creating a situation where withdrawal will be difficult or impossible.

By using the information in this text, the practitioner can help many of the endocrine disorders seen in daily clinical practice. If these methods are used in lieu of hormone replacement therapy, the patient can look forward to good health without the side effects that may accompany conventional endocrine treatments.

Afterword

As Sherlock Holmes said, "It is my business to know what others do not." In integrative endocrinology, it is necessary for the practitioner to adopt this motto.

Read, study, question. The doctor's understanding of the individual case and the analysis of the patient's symptoms is more important than the lab report. As an example, to run a thyroid-stimulating hormone (TSH) test on a person with several hypothyroid symptoms and pronounce him or her well if the test is in the normal range is not careful practice. This approach is used every day even though the textbooks of endocrinology warn against it. As an integrative endocrinologist, you must correlate the symptoms and functions of not just one gland but perhaps several. Thus, having more than one modality is important for the treatment to be effective and while changing the treatment course of an endocrine disorder.

Be attentive during the journey, but keep your eye on the goal of healing. The author will be happy to hear your experience with integrative endocrinology.

Appendix
Twenty-four Hour Urine Hormone Profile

Sex Hormones: Left

Adrenal (Corticosteroids) Hormones: Right

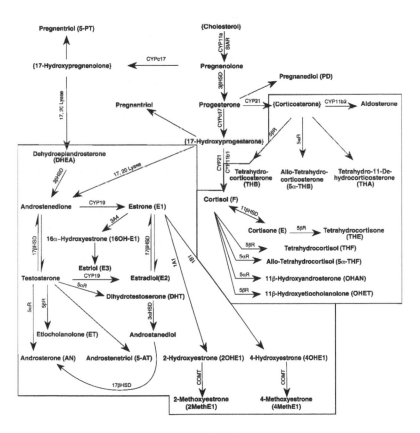

© 2009 Rhein Consulting Laboratories

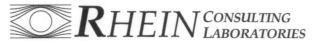

Frank J. Nordt, Ph.D., Director
4475 SW Scholls Ferry Road • Suite 101
Portland, Oregon 97225 USA
Tel: (503) 292-1988
www.rheinlabs.com

Biosynthesis and Metabolism of Steroid Hormones as Produced in the Ovaries, Testes and Adrenals

In the female, Estradiol (E2) is the major biologically active hormone, whereas it is Testosterone (T) in the male. Compounds in brackets {} are intermediates not assayed in urine. Progesterone(P) is metabolized to Pregnanediol (PD) in the liver. P is not normally excreted in urine in measurable quantities and Pregnanediol (PD) as measured in urine reflects Progesterone levels both sensitively and accurately.

Estrogen Metabolism:

1A1: Cytochrome p450 1A1 (CYP1A1)

1B1: Cytochrome p450 1B1 (CYP1B1)

3A4: Cytochrome p450 3A4 (CYP3A4)

COMT: Catechol-O-Methyl-transferase

Enzymatic Steps:

3βHSD:
  3 - beta - Hydroxysteroid dehydrogenase

5αR: 5 - alpha - Reductase

5βR: 5 - beta - Reductase

11βHSD:
  11 - beta - Hydroxysteroid dehydrogenase

17βHSD :
  17 - beta - Hydroxysteroid dehydrogenase

17,20 Lyase: 17,20 - Desmolase

CYP11a: Cholesterol side chain cleavage

StAR: Steroidogenic acute regulatory protein

CYP11b1: 11 - beta - Hydroxylase

CYP11b2: 18 - Oxidase

CYPc17: 17 - alpha - Hydroxylase

CYP19: Aromatase

CYP21: 21 - Hydroxylase

Definitions of the Components of the Twenty-four Hour Urine Hormone Profile

11 β-Hydroxy Androstenedione is an adrenal androgen derived mainly from the hydroxylation of **androstenedione**. Because 11 β-Hydroxylase is an enzyme present only in the adrenal, 11 β-Hydroxy Androstenedione can be used to distinguish adrenal and ovarian sources of androgen overproduction. Hirsute females with an adrenal source of overandrogenization exhibit elevated levels of 11 β-Hydroxy Androstenedione, whereas ovarian disorders, including polycystic ovarian disease, produce normal levels. Hypogonadal males frequently have elevated levels of 11 β-Hydroxy Androstenedione.

Aldosterone is an adrenal hormone produced by the zona glomerulosa. It is produced from pregnenolone and progesterone. Aldosterone causes retention of sodium and chlorine and elimination of potassium and hydrogen. Aldosterone maintains blood pressure and blood volume. Sodium depletion causes aldosterone levels to increase.

Androstenediol (D-5 Androstenediol) Androstenediol is an androgen produced primarily from reversible conversion of **dehydroepiandrosterone**. It is converted peripherally to **testosterone**. Both the adrenal and gonads produce androstenediol. The gonadal contribution in the male is about 90%, whereas the adrenal is the major source for females.

Androstenedione (D-4 Androstenedione) Androstenedione is an androgen originating from both the adrenal gland and the gonads. It is produced metabolically from both 17-Hydroxy-progesterone and **dehydroepiandrosterone**. It is metabolized to **estrone** and reversibly converted to **testosterone**.

Cortisol (Compound F, Hydrocortisone) Cortisol is the major corticosteroid produced by the adrenal gland. It is reversibly converted to **cortisone**. ACTH controls cortisol production. Urine cortisol levels are very elevated in Cushing's disease. Estrogens, Hyperthyroidism, ACTH, and Corticotropin Releasing Hormone stimulate cortisol levels. Cortisol is suppressed by chronic renal failure, nephrotic syndrome, starvation, and Dexamethasone.

Cortisone (Compound E)   is a Corticosteroid converted reversibly from cortisol by the adrenal gland, liver, and in peripheral tissues. Cortisone has only weak glucocorticoid activity.

Dehydroepiandrosterone (DHEA)   is a 17-ketosteroid produced primarily by the adrenal gland. It is reversibly converted to Dehydroepiandrosterone-Sulfate and to **androstenediol**. It is also converted to **androstenedione**. DHEA is one of the first androgens to increase significantly at the onset of adrenarche, which is the onset of the production of steroids before age eight. Levels increase throughout puberty until adulthood. In females, levels drop off sharply after menopause. DHEA may help separate adrenal causes from gonadal causes of overandrogenization.

Estradiol (E2)   (17b-Estradiol) is one of three estrogens derived from metabolism of **testosterone** and converted reversibly to **estrone**. Estradiol is the most potent estrogen. Postmenopausal women produce very little glandular estradiol. The levels found usually come from peripheral conversion of testosterone.

Estriol (E3)   is one of three estrogens along with **estrone** and **estradiol**. During pregnancy, estriol is the most abundant estrogen present with significant quantities formed from **dehydroepiandrosterone** derivatives. In males and in non-pregnant females, estriol is found in very low concentrations.

Estrone (E1)   is one of the three estrogens derived from metabolism of **androstenedione** and converted rapidly and reversibly to **estradiol**. Estrone has only weak estrogenic properties. Aging and obesity are two major factors controlling production of estrone. Postmenopausal women produce very little glandular estrone. The levels found usually come from peripheral conversion of androstenedione. Estrone levels are higher in the luteal phase.

Etiocholanolone   is one of the three major 17-ketosteroids together with Androsterone and **dehydroepiandrosterone**. It is derived primarily from **androstenedione** although it can also be produced from other androgens.

Pregnanediol-3-Glucuronide   is metabolized primarily from **progesterone**. Patients with luteal phase defect have significantly lower levels during the first few days of the luteal phase. Levels of Pregnanediol-3-Glucuronide increase steadily in pregnancy. Increased levels may indicate the onset of endometrial cancer.

Progesterone   is a Progestin produced primarily from enzymatic metabolism of Pregnenolone. It is enzymatically converted to 17-Hydroxy Progesterone and 11-Deoxycorticosterone. Both the gonads and the adrenal glands secrete it. It is bound to Cortisol Binding Globulin and Albumin, but a small percentage is present in the "free" bioactive form. Progesterone is responsible for cellular changes in the cervix, vagina, and uterus. Levels are lowest in the follicular phase and increase rapidly following the luteal surge. There is a significant increase during pregnancy.

Testosterone In males, Luteinizing Hormone controls production of the majority of testosterone by control of the Leydig cells. In females, most of the testosterone is of adrenal origin. It is produced by metabolism of **androstenedione** and **androstenediol**. It is converted to **estradiol**, dihydrotestosterone, androsterone, and **etiocholanolone**. Testosterone is responsible for much of the 17-ketosteroids found in the urine. Testosterone is responsible for development of secondary sex characteristics in males including external genitalia, growth of facial hair and pubic hair.

Tetrahydroaldosterone (THA) Elevated levels of Aldosterone are usually found in patients with primary aldosteronism, however normal levels usually occur in patients with essential hypertension.

Tetrahydrocorticosterone (THB) Measurements of urine tetrahydro-corticosterone give an accurate assessment of Corticosterone production and clearance.

Tetrahydrocortisol (THF) Measurement of tetrahydrocortisol gives an accurate assessment of cortisol production and clearance.

Tetrahydrocortisone (THE) Measurements of urine tetrahydrocortisone give an accurate assessment of **cortisone** production and clearance.

Thyroxine (T4) is a thyroid hormone produced by coupling of two Diiodo Tyrosines. It is metabolized by mono-deiodination to produce **triiodothyronine** and Reverse Triiodothyronine. Levels of Urine Thyroxine are elevated in hyperthyroidism and in Graves' disease.

Triiodothyronine (T3) is a thyroid hormone produced by coupling of Monoiodo and Diiodo Tyrosines. It is also produced by mono-deiodination of **thyroxine**. Levels of Urine Triiodothyronine are elevated in hyperthyroidism. In Graves' disease, they are elevated to a greater extent than **thyroxine**. Patients with T3 Thyrotoxicosis have elevated Urine T3 but normal T4 levels. Levels are also elevated during pregnancy. In primary hypothyroid patients, Urine Triiodothyronine levels are suppressed to about one-half that of normal.

Resources

abebooks.com
Many of the old texts mentioned in this book are available here

Apothacure
4001 McEwen Rd. #100
Dallas, TX 75244
800-969-6601
www.apothecure.com
Many of the injectable products in this book are available here

Dinshah Health Society
P.O. Box 707
Malaga, NJ 08328
Color therapy information and books

Dr. Ron's Ultra-Pure®
48 Sperry Road
Watertown, CT 06795
877-472-8701
www.DrRons.com
Supplements, fish oil, butter oil, freeze dried glands from New Zealand

Hahnemann Laboratories
1940 Fourth St.
San Rafael, CA 94901
415-451-6978
Excellent source for high quality homeopathic remedies

Health Concerns
8001 Capwell Drive
Oakland, CA 94621

800-233-9355
www.healthconcerns.com
American made Chinese herbal formulas

Heel
Albuquerque, NM 87123
800-621-7644
Combination homeopathics including injectable from the Reckewig formulas

Herb Pharm®
P.O. Box 116
Williams, OR 97544
800-348-4372
www.herb-pharm.com
Western herbal tinctures

International Foundation for Nutrition and Health
3963 Mission Blvd.
San Diego, CA 92109
858-488-8932
Information and books of Royal Lee, Westin Price, Melvin Page, and Francis
Pottenger

Lhasa OMS®
230 Libbey Parkway
Weymouth, MA 02189
800-722-8775
www.LhasaOMS.com
Acupuncture needles, charts, books, Japanese medical supplies

NuHerbs®
3820 Penniman Avenue
Oakland, CA 94619
800-233-4307
www.nuherb.com
Chinese patent medicines, single herbs, American-made Chinese patent
medicines

Shentrition
Dr. Stephen Rogers
P.O. Box 138
Ronan, MT 59864

866-497-7436
www.shentrition.com

Standard Process Inc.®
1200 West Royal Lee Drive
P.O. Box 904
Palmyra, WI 53156-0904
800-848-5061
www.standardprocess.com
Whole food supplements, gland products, Dr. Royal Lee's Protomorphology

Bibliography

Abraham, G.E. (2005) "The Wolff–Chaikoff Effect: Crying Wolf," *The Original Internist*, 12(3): 112–118.

Abrams, Albert (1910) *Spondylotherapy*. San Francisco, CA: Philopolis Press.

Addison, Thomas ([1885] 1980) *Disease of the Supra-Renal Capsules*. Birmingham, AL: The Classics of Medicine Library.

American Medical Association (1916) *New and Unofficial Remedies*. Detroit, MI: American Medical Association.

American Medical Association (1946) *New and Unofficial Remedies*. Detroit, MI: American Medical Association.

Arroyo, C.F. (1924) "Asthencoria," *Med. Jour. and Rec.*, Jan. 2, cxix, p. 25.

Barker, Lewellys (1922) *Endocrinology and Metabolism*. New York: Appleton & Co., p. 22.

Bellavite, Paolo and Andrea Signorini (1995) *Homeopathy: A Frontier in Medical Science*. Berkeley, CA: North Atlantic.

Bensky, Dan (1981) *Acupuncture: A Comprehensive Text*. Chicago: Eastland Press, p. 46.

Besredka, A.M. (1909) *De L'Anaphylaxie. Sixieme memoire de l'anaphylaxie lactique*. Ann. Institute Pastuer 23: 166.

Bicknell, F. and F. Prescott (1953) *The Vitamins in Medicine*. London: William Heinmann Medical Books.

Bone, Kerry and Simon Mills (2000) *Principles and Practice of Phytotherapy*. London: Churchill Livingstone.

Braunwald, E., Faugi, A.S., Kasper, D.L., Hauser, S.L., Longo, D.L. and Jameson, T.L. (2001) *Harrison's Principles of Internal Medicine*. New York: McGraw-Hill.

Brown-Sequard (1889) "The Effects Produced on Man by Subcutaneous Injections of a Liquid Obtained from the Testicles of Animals," *The Lancet*, July 20: 105–107.

Chen, Chi-Ling, Weiss, N.S., Newcomb, P., Barlow, W. and White, E. (2002). "Hormone Replacement Therapy in Relation to Breast Cancer," *Journal of the American Medical Association*, 287 (6): 734–741.

Christopher, John (1976) *School of Natural Healing*. Springville, UT: Christopher Publications.

Coulter, Harris (1973) *Divided Legacy: The Conflict Between Homeopathy and the American Medical Association*. Berkley, CA: North Atlantic Books.

Cowan, Eliot (1995) *Plant Spirit Medicine*. Newberg, OR: Swan Raven & Company.

Cushing, H. (1911) *The Pituitary Body and Its Disorders*. Philadelphia: J.B. Lippincott Company, pp. 315–316.

Cushing, Harvey (1921) "Disorders of the Pituitary Gland Retrospective and Prophetic," *Journal of the American Medical Association*, 76 (25): 1721–1726.

Day, C. (1995) *The Homeopathic Treatment of Beef and Dairy Cattle*. Beaconsfield, England: Beaconsfield, p. 120.

Deadman, Peter (2001) *A Manual of Acupuncture*. Hove, England: Journal of Chinese Medicine Publications.

Dinshah, Darius (1985) *Let There Be Light*. Malaga, NJ: Dinshah Health Society.

Dinshah, Ghadiali P. (1939) *Spectro-Chrome Metery Encyclopaedia*. Malaga, NJ: Spectro-Chrome Institute.

Dorland's Illustrated Medical Dictionary (2003). Philadelphia PA: Saunders.

Dosch, Peter (1984) *Manual of Neural Therapy According to Huneke*. Heidelberg: Karl F. Haug.

Federman, D. (2003) "The Endocrine Patient" in *Williams Textbook of Endocrinology*, 10th ed. Philadelphia, PA: W.B. Saunders, p. 15.

Fishbein, M. (ed.) (1948) Book Review: *Protomorphology, Journal of the American Medical Association*, 138 (ii), September–December: 856.

Fratkin, J.P. (2001) *Chinese Herbal Medicines*. Shva Publications.

Guyton, Arthur and John E. Hall (2000) *Textbook of Medical Physiology*. Philadelphia, PA: W.B. Saunders.

Hahnemann, Samuel ([1842] 1996) *The Organon of the Medical Art*, 6th ed., edited and annotated by Wenda Brewster O'Reilly. Redmond, WA: Birdcage Books.

Harrower, Henry R. (1917) *The Internal Secretions in Practical Medicine*. Chicago: Chicago Medical Book Co.

Harrower, Henry R. (1922) *Practical Organotherapy*. Glendale, CA: The Harrower Laboratory.

Hensley, Kenneth, Benaksas, E.J., Bolli, R., Grammas, P., Hamdheydari, L. Mou, S., Pye, Q. N., Stoddard, M. F., Wallis, G., Williamson, K. S., West, M., Wechter, W.J. and Floyd, R.A. (2004) "New Perspectives on Vitamin E: Gamma Tocopherol, and Carboxythydroxychroman Metabolites in Biology and Medicine," *Free Radical Biology and Medicine*, 36 (1): 1–15.

Hertoghe, T. (2006) *The Hormone Handbook*. Surrey, UK: International Medical Publications.

Hochberg, Ze'ev, Pacak, K. and Chrousos, G.P. (2003) "Endocrine Withdrawal Syndromes," *Endocrine Reviews*, 24: 523–538.

Hutchens, Alma (1973) *Indian Herbology of North America*. Windsor, Ontario: Merco.

Jarvis, D.C. (1958) *Folk Medicine*. New York: Henry Holt & Co.

Jensen, Bernard (1983) *Iridology: The Science and Practice in the Healing Arts*, Vol. II. Escondido, CA: Bernard Jensen.

Julian, O.A. (1979) *Materia Medica of New Homeopathic Remedies*. Beaconsfield, England: Beaconsfield, p. 234.

Klenijnen, J., Knipschild, P. and Riet, G. (1991) "Clinical Trials of Homeopathy," *British Medical Journal*, 302 (6772): 316–332.

Lee, J.R. (1999) *What your Doctor May not Tell you About Premenopause. Natural versus Synthetic Hormones*. New York: Warner Books, p. 34.

Lee, Royal (1950) *The Battlefront for Better Nutrition*. Reprint No. 30-E. Milwaukee, WI: Lee Foundation for Nutritional Research.

Lee, Royal (2003) *Lectures of Dr. Royal Lee*, Vol. 2. Fort Collins, CO: Selene River Press.

Manaka, Y. and Stephen Birch (1995) *Chasing the Dragon's Tail*. Taos, NM: Paradigm Publications.

McKeon, Richard (ed.) (1941) "Metaphysics," in *The Basic Works of Aristotle*. New York: Random House.

Merck & Co. (1934) *Merck Manual*. Rahway, NJ: Merck & Co., p. 117.

Murray (1891) "Note on the Treatment of Myxoedema by Hypodermic Injection of an Extract of the Thyroid Gland of a Sheep," *British Medical Journal*, London, II: 796.

Needham, Joseph (1980) *Celestial Lancets*. Cambridge, England: University Press, p. 269.

Netter, Frank (1965) *The Endocrine System*. New York: Ciba Pharmaceutical Company.

Niehans, Paul (1960) *Introduction to Cellular Therapy*. New York: Pageant Books.

Nogier, Paul (1972) *Treatise of Auriculotherapy*. Moulins-les-Metz, France: Maissonneuve.

Palmer, D.D. (1910) *The Chiropractor's Adjuster: The Science, Art, and Philosophy of Chiropractic*. Portland, OR: Portland Printing House.

Pliny ([72] 1938) *Natural History*, trans. H. Rackman. Boston, MA: Harvard University Press.

Ramakrishnan, A.U. (2001) Personal communication with the author, Denver, CO.

Sahelian, Ray (1996) *DHEA: A Practical Guide*. Garden City Park, NY: Avery.

Sajous, C. (1922) *The Internal Secretions and the Principles of Medicine*. Philadelphia, PA: F.A. Davis.

Sankaran, Rajan (1997) *The Soul of Remedies*. Bombay, India: Homeopathic Medical Publishers.

Schmid, F., and J. Stein (1967) *Cell Research and Cellular Therapy*. Thoune, Switzerland: Ott.

Selye, Hans (1947) *Textbook of Endocrinology*. Acta Endocrinologica, University de Montreal, Canada, p. 41.

Shakespeare, William (1601) *Hamlet*, Act 1, Scene 2.

Shumaker, Sally A., Legault, C., Rapp, S.R., Thal, L., Wallace, R.B., Ockene, J.K., Hendrix, S.L., Jones, B.N., III, Assaf, A.R., Jackson, R.D., Kotchen, J.M., Wassertheil-Smoller, S. and Wactawski-Winder, J. (2003) "Estrogen Plus Progestin and the Incidence of Dementia and Mild Cognitive Impairment in Postmenopausal Women: A Randomized Controlled Trial," *Journal of the American Medical Association*, 289 (20): 2651–2662.

Spring, Charles (1921) *Treatise on Organotherapy*. Chicago: published by the author.

Travell, Janet (1983) *Myofascial Pain and Dysfunction: The Trigger Point Manual*. Baltimore, MD: Williams & Wilkins.

Vithoulkas, George (1980) *The Science of Homeopathy*. New York: Grove Press, p.162.

Voll, Reinhold (1978) *Topographic Positions of the Measurement Points in Electro-Acupuncture Text*, Vol. 1. Uelzen, Germany: Medizinish Literarische Verlagsgesellschaft MBH, pp. 75–76.

Weiner, Howard (ed.) (2004) *Oral Tolerance*. Annals of the New York Academy of Sciences, New York.

Wells, H.G. and Osborne, T.B. (1911) "The Biological Reactions of the Vegetable Proteins, I. Anaphylaxis," *Journal of Infectious Diseases*, 8: 66.

Williams Textbook of Endocrinology (2003) 10th ed., Philadelphia, PA: W.B. Saunders.

Wolf, William (1940) *Endocrinology in Modern Practice*. Philadelphia, PA: W.B. Saunders.

Yang JiZhou (1981) *Great Compendium of Acupuncture (Jin Jiu Da Jing)*. Taiwan, p. 111. (In Chinese.)

Yen, P. (2002) *Hormone Resistance and Hypersensitivity States*. Philadelphia, PA: Lippincott Williams & Wilkins.

Reading List

Beinfield, H., and E. Korngold (1991) *Between Heaven and Earth*. New York: Ballantine Books.

Bensky, Dan (1981) *Acupuncture: A Comprehensive Text*. Chicago: Eastland Press, p. 46.

Deadman, Peter (2001) *A Manual of Acupuncture*. Hove, England: Journal of Chinese Medicine Publications.

For a full discussion of the historical influence of acupuncture and its eventual movement into all cultural areas of the world, see:

Needham, Joseph (1980) *Celestial Lancets*. Cambridge, England: Cambridge University Press.

Schmid, F., and J. Stein (1967) *Cell Research and Cellular Therapy*. Thoune, Switzerland: Ott Publishers.

Neihans, P. (1960) *Introduction to Cellular Therapy*. New York: Pageant Books.

Dosch, Peter (1984) *Manual of Neural Therapy according to Huneke*. Heidelberg: Karl F. Haug Publishers.

Dosch, Mathias (1985) *Illustrated Atlas of the Techniques of Neural Therapy with Local Anesthetics*. Heidelberg: Karl F. Haug Publishers.

For additional herbal information or to research the effects of herbs mentioned in this text, see:

Bone, Kerry, and Simon Mills (2000) *Principles and Practice of Phytotherapy*. London, England: Churchill Livingstone.

Hutchens, Alma (1973) *Indian Herbology of North America*. Windsor, Ontario: Merco.

Christopher, John (1976) *School of Natural Healing*. Springville, UT: Christopher Publications.

Weiss, Rudolf Fritz (n.d) *Herbal Medicine*. Beaconsfield, England: Beaconsfield Publishers.

Jensen, Bernard (1978) *Nature Has a Remedy*. Escondido, CA. Bernard Jensen Publishing.

Any U.S. or British Pharmacopia printed before 1920 or, preferably, 1900 as almost all the remedies contained in these books are whole herb in nature and not created by synthetic means or complex extracting processes that would change the properties of the complete herb.

Amber, R.B. (1964) *Color Therapy*. Calcutta, India: Firma KLM Private Limited.

Babbitt, E. (1967) *The Principles of Light and Color*. New Hyde Park, NY: University Books.

Index

About the Author

Dr. Donald R. Beans, a native Montana, began working in the medical field as an aide in the emergency department in 1973. Dr. Beans is a registered nurse with a degree from Montana State University, 1978. He studied acupuncture at many schools and with various teachers leading to Montana licensure in 1980 and starting a private practice in Missoula. He earned national board certification in acupuncture in 1985 from the National Commission for the Certification of Acupuncture and Oriental Medicine; he is also a certified classical homeopath.

Dr. Beans was a teaching associate of Dr. Bernard Jensen for 10 years, 1983–1993. They presented one-week seminars on nutrition and wellness. Under the watchful eye of Dr. Jensen, Dr. Beans earned a doctor of philosophy degree in iridology and nutrition from the University of Health Science in Honolulu, Hawaii.

Dr. Beans joined the Endocrine Society in 2003 and attended the course *Clinical Endocrinology* at Harvard Medical School.

Dr. Beans is currently in private practice in Bigfork, Montana, and in an integrative medical practice, The Bridge Medical Center, in Whitefish Montana.

Milton Keynes UK
Ingram Content Group UK Ltd.
UKHW031151141024
449569UK00024B/893